Variations of Normal

The Labors of Love

Kinsey Phifer

Copyright © 2021

Variations of Normal: The Labors of Love

Kinsey Phifer

This book is not intended to be used as a substitute for medical advice from a licensed physician. Please consult your healthcare provider to address your specific health needs.

Design Services: Deborah King
Author Photo: Michael David Imagery

ISBN: 978-1-7374244-0-6 (Print)

To my two children.
Thank you for teaching me the valuable lessons of motherhood.

Author's Note

The stories from the individuals in this book were obtained with permission. In order to protect each individual's anonymity, no names have been used. The following stories do not necessarily reflect my own opinions on the topics shared in this book. These stories are not intended to be a substitute for medical advice of a licensed physician.

The events and quotes in my own story were documented and recalled to the best of my memory. I do not believe there is a 'perfect' way to birth; however, I believe every individual has the right to respectful care and informed choices.

Contents

Preface

"It's just a variation of normal."

That's what I was told when I found out my first baby was breech. I was told this again when I found out my uterus is heart shaped. It's all just a variation of normal. There are so many variations of normal in pregnancy, birth, parenthood and life. No two people will look at the same experience the same way. What one person finds empowering, the next may find traumatizing. Some might feel a combination of both.

When I started this book, I had no idea where it would go. I started writing it after my second child was born via another unplanned cesarean. Originally it was an outlet to help process both of my birth experiences and even some other past traumas. My hope was for people to better understand my point of view on how these experiences affected me.

Somewhere along the way, I invited others to share their experiences, and it became so much more. There are so many powerful stories here. As mothers we tend to feel alone, when in reality so many feel the same way. Not every story will resonate with you, and that's okay. These stories may be triggering to some, but they are experiences worth sharing. I hope we can all hold space for each other and listen respectfully. None of your feelings are wrong.

These are all variations of normal.

Part One

Their Stories

This book features over 100 different people sharing their experiences. It shows how pregnancy, giving birth and parenthood have a deep impact on all of us. Some of these stories are happy, some are sad, and some will make you uncomfortable. Every story has a lesson. My hope is that people will read this with an open mind and walk in someone else's shoes for just one moment without judgment.

These are stories that need to be heard. I can only hope I'm honoring all of the people who contributed their experiences with this book. I hope that they feel heard and validated. I hope that in reading these stories, you do too.

Pregnancy

There are so many emotions at play when you find out you're pregnant. Any feeling is possible, ranging from excited, scared, sad, relieved, angry, and more. Chances are if you are feeling it, someone else has too. There are few other things in life that are as complex as the emotions that come with pregnancy.

You Truly Know Them

I was excited when I found out I was pregnant. I was told I would be lucky to ever have any children due to my endometriosis, and I got two! I hated pregnancy, though. I was sick, throwing up most of the pregnancies. The best part was feeling them kick and wiggle around inside my tummy. Everything about that part was amazing because you are really the only one who truly knows them at this point. You start to find their routines and what they like and don't like before anyone else.

He Saved Me

I didn't want children at all, and when I found out I was accidentally pregnant, I felt AWFUL. I felt like someone besides me deserved it more and that I shouldn't be excited because I didn't ask for it. But he really ended up saving me. It's totally normal to feel highs and lows during pregnancy. If I'd known what I was feeling back then was depression, I probably would have asked for some intervention when I was pregnant. It got to the point where I didn't feel any joy the day he was born, and if I would have known that I had depression, I would have done something before then. Your feelings are TOTALLY normal! My baby was an accident and we never wanted kids. I relate to the lack of excitement especially in regards to the way people "normally" feel. Your feelings, or lack thereof, are normal. I love my boy, but it definitely took some time.

5

A Walking Zombie

My first pregnancy was great. My second one was a little harder. I had a really hard time connecting with him because I experienced infertility and miscarriages for almost three years prior. My current pregnancy has been very rough. I'm a walking zombie and really sick. I just feel overall like I'm struggling and not being the best wife/ mom I can be. It's hard to remind myself that this isn't forever and I'm doing my best. This pregnancy has been the hardest mentally and physically, and I'm only 12 weeks.

I Was in Shock

During the first trimester, I was struggling. I'm sure it had a lot to do with the pandemic and lack of human interaction. When I went to the OBGYN appointment, I thought it would be the happiest moment. My husband was crying, and it was special, but I didn't feel anything. I felt a lot of shame about this. It scared me because I felt like there was something wrong with me. I wanted to get pregnant eventually, but I had been struggling with some health stuff that I wanted to figure out before getting pregnant. So there was a lot of frustration that we got pregnant when we did. Of course I wanted this baby, but I had been wrestling with a lot of depressive thoughts and lack of interest in most things at that time.

It's as if I went into shock and felt numb. My husband is always very supportive, but I wasn't voicing my side of things because I felt ashamed. I just felt super low most of the time. It was deeper than just being tired. Everything felt daunting, like doing the dishes or laundry or anything really. When I made myself get outside to walk, that always helped, but the second I got back in the house, I felt depressed again. I had feelings of loneliness, like things didn't matter, bitterness, and I was more irritable than I've ever been. I felt that something was wrong when I was on the phone with my dad and he said something like, "These are such exciting times," and I just sort of felt nothing. Things are going better now and I'm excited to meet my little one!

Your Heart Grows

I was mad when I found out I was pregnant with our second baby. Like furious. I wasn't ready. We just lost our house in a fire and everything I owned was in one room in my mom's house. I already had a baby. I was afraid. I didn't think I could love someone as much as I loved my first child.

I didn't think I could be as good of a mom to two babies as I was to one. I worried about how I was going to mess them up. I didn't know how we were going to afford it. I was over it after about an hour because I realized how lucky I was to be alive and I had my family. My mom just laughed at me and said, "Of course you will love this second baby." Your heart grows with each baby you create!

Mixed Emotions

I felt robbed of the time I had left before starting a family. I felt sad because I knew it was the end of my career. I always knew I would stay home with my babies. I felt worried about connecting with our baby if it was a girl because of my broken relationship with my mom. But I also felt excited because having babies was my dream!

I Never Thought I Could Get Pregnant

I was shocked when I found out I was pregnant since I was told I was infertile. I was told that I couldn't get pregnant, let alone carry to term, and my chances were higher for miscarriage or stillbirth. I never thought I'd be able to get pregnant again, let alone maintain the pregnancy. I was 11 weeks along when I found out.

Real Life Learning Experience

The first time I found out I was pregnant, I was 24 and in my first marriage. We were trying to get pregnant, but it was a bit different for us because my partner already had a daughter from another relationship. To be honest, I didn't realize how difficult my first pregnancy would be since it was seen as unwanted by my partner's side of the family. This was something that would later become a burden on our marriage and eventually lead to one of the major reasons we are no longer together. I was also in school at the time and learning how to juggle being a stepmom to a little girl whose mother had walked out on her. Throughout my whole pregnancy I struggled with my role as step parent and becoming a first time parent to my own child. I never felt I was doing anything right for my stepdaughter in the eyes of my in-laws. I often felt that my unborn child was seen as an issue by his side of the family.

Jump 10 years later and I'm pregnant again with my second child and in my second marriage. His side of the family is much more mature about our pregnancy and is more accepting of our child. He has a child from another marriage who is four and it's a little easier this time around because her mother is still involved and is HERE. I don't feel like I am responsible for another person's child and need to fill a role that I can't or should not be required to do. I feel pretty grateful that God has given me a second chance at having a blended family and this time with more mature adults who actually know how to be parents. I guess the only thing that I regret is that I waited so long to try and find happiness in my first marriage, when I should have seen the warning signs from the start and left early on. But I am glad that I have my wonderful first born child from that marriage and some real life learning experience.

I Was Ecstatic

Despite the fact that I was 18 years old and not in a committed relationship, I was ecstatic to find out I was pregnant. I was so happy to have someone to love and who would love me. I had an overwhelming love for my child. I knew I would love them but just how strongly, I had no idea there was a love that large.

You Push Yourself

I was scared. I guess I knew my partner wasn't fit to be a parent so I knew I was going to be on my own. You find out how strong you are. I thought I was tough before but now I'm "mommy tough." You push yourself more than you ever will in life just to make sure they have everything they need. Time stood still, and for once in my life I knew I was right where I needed to be.

Blessed

The first time I found out I was pregnant, I freaked out as I was only 19 and taking birth control pills. The second time, I was overjoyed as we had been trying for two and a half years. The third time I was angry because our second one had just turned one, and I didn't want them that close. The fourth time I felt blessed to have one last one.

Entirely Different Role

I was 29 when I "suspected" I was pregnant with my first. I talked myself out of my condition by convincing myself that it was probably diabetes or another ailment. I did, however, go to my doctor appointment. She congratulated me and said, "You'll be fine!" I was so freaked out. This would be an entirely different role for us. We both had concentrated on our jobs and getting ahead for our first 5 years together.

I craved grapefruit, bell peppers and Mexican food. I read everything I could find about pregnancy and labor. We went to Lamaze class with couples who were markedly younger than we were. I enjoyed my pregnancy, but the heart burn was ridiculous the entire time. We even stayed home on New Years Eve because I felt like a fire breathing dragon. I took remarkable care of myself and did all the right things. I was rocking the preggers thing!

The Most Joyous Moment

I was in awe. We had been trying for a little while, and when I finally got that positive, it was the most joyous moment of my life! This is really happening!

Every Emotion

We had been trying to get pregnant for 10 years and had two miscarriages. I think I felt every emotion in the book. After two miscarriages, I was convinced I was going to have another this time around. When we found out we were having three babies, I was not sure if they would all make it. I had to quit reading baby books because they only stressed me out telling me everything that could go wrong with multiple births. But the further along I got, the more excited I got about having my babies. Then I ended up on bed rest and there was a lot of stress with that. Health wise, I felt really good even with my body doing all these weird things.

I Wouldn't Change a Thing

I was in denial. I had been on birth control for 5 years and I took a Plan B after that one instance. I couldn't believe it happened and never ever dreamt of being a mom. I was depressed for the first 7 months. I started to accept it when my belly was huge, after my baby shower, and once I put the nursery together. The most surprising thing is how much you can truly love someone. My son gives me the most motivation ever. My pregnancy wasn't planned, and his birth didn't go as planned, but I'm more than happy he is here and that I am his mother. I wouldn't change a thing.

I Consider Myself Lucky

My first pregnancy I was absolutely terrified. I was young, not married, but in a stable relationship. It happened out of nowhere. It blindsided us. My second pregnancy we fought so hard for. I had a miscarriage and it took what seemed like forever to get pregnant. I felt like I was failing after getting pregnant so easily the first time. When we finally found out, I just remember crying tears of joy, but having that constant worry something was going to happen.

With my third pregnancy, I was feeling really off. I thought it could be my thyroid so I made a doctor's appointment, but I thought, "Ya know, just in case I'm going to take a test." Positive! I remember texting my husband a picture, and we were both speechless because our daughter was freshly one and it was a little too soon. We finally got our heads wrapped around the fact we would have three kids, then we found out at our eight week ultrasound it was TWINS!

I had very easy pregnancies for the most part, so I consider myself lucky. My first pregnancy, I was barely sick up until the end when he was pushing all on my insides. With the second and third, I had morning sickness the entire pregnancy. It was like clockwork in the morning. Once I got it out of my system, I could go on with my day.

Felt Like a Dream

When I found out I was pregnant, I felt surprised and nervous. I felt like I wasn't near ready to be a parent. Honestly, I felt like it was a weird dream that I just kept having, especially since I didn't actually start to look pregnant until about 36 weeks.

So Exhausted

I was going through a very stressful time in my life stretching myself too thin and feeling very run down. I was staying up too late working on a project for my husband and was having a very difficult time having energy to accomplish everything I needed to get done. I felt so sick and thought maybe I had Mono or some horrible illness. I hardly ever go to the doctor but finally had enough and couldn't seem to figure out why I was so exhausted. Nothing tasted right and I was nauseous. I thought maybe I had a bladder infection because I had to pee all the time. I made an appointment at the doctor's office and was telling them my symptoms.

They had me do a urine test. The nurse came back into the room with the results and said, "The doctor ran the test three times, and each time the test came back positive." I looked at her dumbfounded and asked, "Positive for what?" She said, "Well, you're pregnant!" I was shocked! I started to cry with both fear and happiness at the same time. Fear because I was 38 years old, and my husband and I hadn't planned on having another baby. Happiness because I always wanted more children. I felt so dumb since I already had two other children. This was not my first time around the block. I had been so preoccupied that I didn't even notice any missing periods. I wasn't even sure how far along I was. As it turned out, I was already almost three months along!

A Lot of Work

I felt miserable! I was sick, in some way, for almost the entire pregnancy each time. I had nausea day and night for the first trimesters of each pregnancy. I had preterm issues and had to give myself shots for my last pregnancy. Being pregnant was a lot of work for me. I never felt like a glowing mother-to-be.

I Loved It

When I found out I was pregnant, I was extremely happy. Proud. Excited. Relieved. Honestly, I loved being pregnant! It made me happy and excited to be able to create a baby.

The Labors of Love

When starting a family there are many different kinds of labors of love. Some of these labors occur during childbirth, while others are through adoption. It is all hard work. No two stories are the same, just like no two people are the same. Some births go according to plan, while others wind up totally different from how we imagined. Birth can be calm, exciting, dramatic, scary or all of the above!

Our Choices

I think our birth choices ultimately teach us about parenting. As our kids grow, we have to choose what's best for our families and ourselves. Sometimes it will look so different from the next family or our families growing up. And that's perfectly okay.

The Most Incredible Thing I Have Ever Done

I cried like crazy when I found out I was pregnant. I wasn't ready and didn't feel as excited or even that it was real when I saw or heard my baby for the first time. Even when I gave birth to him it wasn't overwhelming love, which is so embarrassing and shameful to me. I had a really hard labor and long delivery. I felt like I didn't know him and I felt like I should. I don't know how to explain it. He and my other two are the most incredible things I have ever done. Love is nothing that can be described, but it doesn't always come instantly.

I Caught My Own Baby

It was a gorgeous Saturday in January, so we opted to detail the van and get the third car seat installed in preparation for our newest arrival. I didn't feel great the rest of the day. My body ached, and I felt I overdid it on the van. I would have the occasional contraction, maybe one every 30 minutes to 2 hours. Around 1:30 a.m. on Sunday, my contraction frequency and intensity suddenly increased. I hung out in the bathroom for about 15 minutes, wondering how I was going to make it through and if it was "time" yet. I decided it might not be a bad idea to call my mom over to watch the boys. Just then, I heard our 20 month old over the baby monitor. I woke my husband up to get him and said he should call my mom, too.

I slowly made my way out to see if he'd had a chance to make the call yet, and he hadn't. Our toddler was needing his daddy to put him back to sleep. I made the call to my mom around 2:00 a.m., just in time to feel the rapid descent of a baby. I realized at that moment that this was happening right now, and we were on our own. We did have a home birth with our second, but that one was planned. We were not planning it with this baby. I was expecting to labor at home in a birth tub, that I was generously loaned, as long as possible. Then we would make the trip to the hospital I work in for the birth. Perfectly laid out plans, right.... I hollered out to my hubby to call 9-1-1 and made my way to the birth tub, where I delivered her head. By this time, my nerves had eased up. I was not only a birthing mother, but also an experienced birth assistant, thinking of all the things that needed to happen. Within a few minutes of the 9-1-1 call, she was born in the water.

I was extra careful to bring her body up slowly to my chest and not let her go back underwater. I knew her transition would be slower since she was born like a mermaid, and within moments she was pink and crying. I just caught my own baby. Wow, what a feeling!

Even the dogs were celebrating, and our 105 lb Golden Pyranese joined me and Baby Girl in the tub. At least her front half joined us in the tub before my husband pulled her out. In her "excitement" she also peed all over the place, including the phone which was still on speaker phone with the 9-1-1 dispatcher. That resulted in hanging up on him, but within minutes our house was filled with firefighters and medics. It was a real BIRTHday party now! Happy, happy birthday, Little Miss. We will not soon forget your arrival. And thank you to the medics who reminded us to snag a few pictures of the occasion. We did end up taking an ambulance ride to the hospital, where I got to see my lovely coworkers and midwife. We really did want to share more of this experience with them. Maybe next time!

A Very Tired Warrior

I have delivered both babies unmedicated. We used Pitocin in both deliveries as well. It is so hard and the biggest mental marathon I've ever experienced. I am astonished each time at what my mind and body can do. I always feel like a warrior afterwards, a very tired warrior. I was very timid with my first because I didn't know what to expect or how to advocate for myself. I was always second guessing my choices. My labor and delivery team was phenomenal and supported me in ways I didn't even know I needed.

I was more confident for my second birth and asked for things I needed without hesitation. My personal growth made me feel more in control. I was also able to conserve more energy throughout labor because I had learned to not tense my whole body during contractions. I also labored in the water this time, which helped immensely. I have never been a crier in big life moments. Everyone expects you to cry when you get engaged, find your wedding dress or see your baby for the first time. I didn't in any of those scenarios. I think when I saw my babies for the first time, I was just so in awe to finally see and hold this little life that was a mystery for so long. It is an overwhelming experience after working so hard for many hours in labor.

Different Each Time

My first birth experience made me mad. The doctor let me go 17 days past my due date, and I was in labor for 39 hours before I demanded a C-section because I had only dilated to 5 cm. I didn't see my first daughter until about four hours after she was born because they knocked me out after my emergency C-section. I never knew I could love someone so much. My second was a planned C-section and it was great!

Felt Like My Body Failed

I was disappointed in my body. I was stuck at 9 cm for five hours and had to have a cesarean section. I just felt like my body failed me when I had been dreaming of this experience for a lifetime. I had a bout of vomiting that resolved after a few hours, but overall, I was surprised at how good I felt despite having a cesarean. I needed no pain medication and I was up and walking five hours later.

We Surprised Ourselves

My first two births were a breeze and I am really lucky. Some will probably glare at me after reading this. I was induced a week early for both pregnancies, due to end of pregnancy high blood pressure. After the Pitocin was started, I had them about 8 hours later and only pushed three times before they were out. I did have epidurals for both and never had any issues.

With my twins, my goal my entire pregnancy was to be able to have them vaginally. I did not want a C-section after having my other two vaginally. I think I mostly was scared about the recovery time and how I would manage my one year old if I had a C-section. My doctor was very optimistic that I could have them vaginally as long as twin A was head down. There was a mix up with one of my appointments one day and I had to see one of her partners. I wasn't wild about the idea but I didn't want to miss more work than I had to. I remember leaving that appointment so upset and mad because he had made a comment about how I "shouldn't get my hopes up because statically most pregnancies with multiples end up with a C-section and it's just safer." I was so mad because baby B had been breech the entire time, but baby A was head down. So I was SURE I would be able to have them vaginally.

I went in a few weeks later at 34 weeks and we did our normal ultrasound and found that Baby A had turned breech. I sat there and cried while my OB just hugged me and said, "I know you're disappointed but don't get discouraged, we will check every time until the day you deliver to make sure he didn't flip back around." I remember being scared to death. I totally blame my OB's partner for baby A turning. He totally jinxed it. I carried my twins to 37 weeks and 3 days, then went in for a scheduled C-section. For the most part it went okay. However, when baby A was taken out he had swallowed a bunch of fluid and was not breathing. I remember laying there helpless and seeing the fear in my husband's face. The nurses kept telling me, "Everything is fine," but clearly it wasn't. I could see how blue he was and I couldn't hear anything. Finally I heard a big cry and I got to see him for two seconds before they rushed him to the NICU. You'd never know it but my bigger twin was my NICU baby. Baby B was born with no problems. He was a little peanut compared to baby A.

I honestly never thought I would have kids and now I have four. I guess what surprised me is how naturally it came. Don't get me wrong, our house is a hot mess most of the time, but we have really surprised ourselves by how well we can contain the chaos.

I Couldn't Wait To Have More Babies

All three of my births were amazing. I loved every second of them. The hospital staff was very helpful if I had any questions and made me feel at ease with everything. All three of my births were quick. With my third, I was a little anxious because my contractions just weren't progressing and my blood pressure was high. Contractions were staying about 10 minutes apart, so the staff asked me if they could add a little Pitocin to help nudge things along. They told me exactly what they were going to do, what should happen, and walked me through everything beforehand so that I could make my decision. They kept an eye on my blood pressure and answered any questions I had about it. After my first birth, I honestly couldn't wait to have more babies just so I could go back there and experience it all again.

Polaroid Picture

Both of my births were emergency C-sections and very scary. With the first one, I had never had surgery before, so it was terrifying. My baby wasn't responding and had to be life-flighted. My first glimpse of him was by a Polaroid picture that a nurse took so I could see him to name him.

No Words To Describe It

The first time giving birth was miserable. I pushed for almost three hours. The second time was kind of scary. I had a C-section four weeks early due to placenta previa. However, seeing my babies for the first time, there's no words to describe the happiness.

We Are Capable

I think the coolest part with my first is that I went in for a check up the day after my due date and the only complaint I had was it felt like I had a gas bubble making me uncomfortable. I had told my doctor that I didn't have any contractions. No pressure or pain. I was SO comfortable. During that exam I found out I was in fact 5 cm dilated and the "gas bubble" was actually contractions because I was in active labor and didn't even know. It was miraculous! My first labor and delivery was all natural and that was so empowering. The adrenaline of everything kept me going and was more motivating than anything. With that delivery, the scariest part was having my water broken. It seems minimal, but with it being my first birth, I had no idea what to expect. That was the only thing that felt out of my control at the time.

My second delivery was also extremely empowering, although I ended up having to have intrathecal pain medicine about 3/4 of the way through labor because of complications with a 9 lb 12 oz baby. We totally had no idea she was that big. The scariest part was when I was on my final push and she turned on the way out. She turned in the birth canal resulting in a shoulder dystocia. So her head was out, but her shoulder was stuck behind my pubic bone. At the time I wasn't really sure what was happening. It was all hands on deck with a nurse on each leg, the doctor to catch the baby and another nurse to put big pressure on my pelvis. I was just told one big push on the count of three.

She was born, with the cord around her neck from turning and just in a matter of those seconds she was blue. They cut the cord and handed her to me and I remember my doctor telling me, "She's okay. I need you to vigorously rub her back." I did just that and then we got our first cries. It was when she cried, that I realized how scary those moments were. They were all very calm and just reassured me. They didn't tell me what was going on at the time to reduce panic. It was all handled very professionally, and I'm so thankful for that.

The biggest lesson from these experiences was to trust in myself. That my body and mind are capable of so many things. We as women (or humans in general) often underestimate what we are capable of both physically and mentally. Labor and delivery taught me a lot about both.

Instant Love

I was lucky both my babies were out in 7 hours start to finish, even though they were 8 and 9 pounds. My doctors were wonderful and always kept me comfy and relaxed as possible. I felt instant love. I never wanted to let either of my babies go. I could have held and snuggled them forever! I still have that issue some nights when all I want to do is curl up with them and snuggle in tight.

It Was a Great Relief

With my first, I was focused on labor and the unknown. With my other two, I knew what to expect and was able to relax and breathe and let my body labor without freaking out. I was much more vocal of my needs and wants to my doctors and nurses. I was exhausted after the births. It was a great feeling of relief, but I became so worried I wasn't feeling enough love or crying like I was supposed to. With my first it felt like I needed time to get to know him. Now I know how I was feeling. With my last two, I knew how much I was going to love them. It was much more calm and a strong feeling of love.

My Husband Was the Best Support

I did research on my doctor and met with him several times before ever getting pregnant. I knew I wanted him as my doctor during birth. I loved the flow of how everything went throughout my labor, even though I stalled. I felt my doctor knew me and was on my side. He listened and assured me along the way and allowed me to do things I wanted to progress. The most empowering thing was the realization of what my body was capable of and the love I had for my husband and the babies. My family's support was amazing and so important! It really made all the difference. My husband was also very supportive and loving.

I wanted to be in the whirlpool tub so badly, but there were a bunch of different reasons why we couldn't use it. First, someone else was using it, and then we were waiting for it to be cleaned. I told my husband I wanted to be in the water. So he got the shower ready and helped me in it. He sat with me and let the water hit my back, rubbing my back at the same time. He kept his forehead on mine and just told me he loved me. He helped me through the contractions. The nurses kept asking him to get me out of the shower, which I just moaned no a million times. He stuck up for me and told them when I was ready I would come out. He was sure to do whatever I needed. He was the best support.

There have even been instances where people make me feel bad for mentioning the good things about my birth by saying, "Oh, well that's good for you," or "Wish everyone had it as easy as you." I am lucky and grateful, but I feel that somehow my experience is not worth hearing. Maybe that's just guilt on my part because I am very lucky for my experiences. I wish everyone could have what I had.

I Was in Denial

My labor was fairly short. I was in denial about it, so I called work and said I'd be in as soon as contractions let up. I went to the hospital at 9:00 a.m. and she was born a little after 1:00 p.m. She had lots of "stork bites" and her little head was pointed. The day after, she bloomed into this beautiful baby with a halo of blonde hair. She held her hands like she was praying. I was in love with this new little person.

My doctor was this amazing man. He was such a calm presence. I chose a natural, unmedicated labor/ delivery. I'm not even certain there was such a thing as an epidural back then. I never wavered from my original plan. My daughter had a perfect APGAR score, so I felt empowered that I'd stuck to my plan.

Walking Bravely Through Trauma

The births of my children were all so scary. I was worrying all the time if they'd survive. It was like walking bravely through trauma, lying there while they cut me open. The first one was on life-support; the second was placed under a breathing hood. I just wanted to hold them, but I wasn't allowed to.

I was so happy with the last three children to be able to hold and nurse them right after the C-section was done. I learned that I didn't have to let the doctor decide everything. I was so afraid of being pressured into a C-section that I didn't go into the ER when I should have. I wish I would have known that I could say no. I ended up with five C-sections!

My Babies Are Completely Different

It was the Saturday before Easter (I was due Easter Sunday, April 21, 2019.) My mom was in Cedar Rapids ready to be there when I went into labor. I woke up Saturday morning about 4:00 a.m. and felt what I thought were contractions. They were mild, though. I told my fiancé, but I told him if they got worse throughout the day I would let him know because he was going to go to work for the day. I was taking my god-daughter and my step-son to an Easter egg hunt with my mom and future mother-in-law. My niece, nephew and future sister-in-law were going to meet us there. My contractions felt like they were getting a little stronger, but it was also my first baby, so it was hard to tell for sure.

After the Easter egg hunt, we went out to eat with everyone. Then we went and hung out at my future in-laws. About 6:00 p.m. I went back to my house and ate dinner. My fiancé went to bed about 8:30 p.m. and I was on the couch. I was starting to get uncomfortable so I told my fiancé, and we went to the hospital. I got checked in and they checked me. I was only 3 cm dilated, so they asked if I wanted to try sitting in the bathtub in the delivery room to see if it progressed by itself, or if I wanted to start Pitocin. I chose the bathtub. After being in there for about 20 minutes I got out.

They checked me again and I was 5 cm. They were able to start hooking me up to everything and put an IV in to calm me down a bit. I was very nervous since it was my first child.

A little while later they asked if I was ready for the epidural and I said yes. I was just about 6 cm at that point. I was a little more relaxed from what they put in my IV so I wasn't in too much pain, but I was still ready for the epidural. They came in and it went fine. I labored throughout the night and didn't really get much sleep. I texted my mom throughout the night. She was at the hotel waiting for me to tell her to come. I only wanted my fiancé and I in the room for our first baby. At 6:00 a.m. they moved the fetal monitor around and checked up on him because I had been in labor awhile, and they didn't want my baby to be in any kind of distress. They told me he was being a stinker in there but also said it was going fine. About 7:30 a.m. they checked me again and told me I was 10 cm and I was ready to push. My fiancé got up right away to come stand by me. At the time there were four other girls in the next few rooms that were all dilated to a 10 and pushing as well, so my doctor was not in my room yet. I pushed two times and then my nurse said, "Okay, hold on we have to wait for the doctor!" With the epidural I wasn't feeling anything so I was okay. They asked if I wanted to feel his head so I reached down and felt it. It was crazy!

Then the doctor came running in, put on her gown and told me to push again and out came my baby at 7:56 a.m. He was super tiny! They put him on my chest and the first thing I said was, "He is so little!" He was 6 lbs 2 oz. They took him shortly after to check him and make sure everything was all good before giving him back to me. He had a little trouble latching, but then he did just fine. Pictures were taken and tears were shed. I had texted my mom and she made her way to the hospital. I told all of our other family members as well. My dad and step-mom were on their way to Cedar Rapids.

After having my baby, he had to have a lot of checkups because he had some temperature issues. His temperature wouldn't stay up, which could have been because he was so little. After multiple checkups and me sitting in the doctor's office for four hours at a time with a heating lamp for him, things got better after a few weeks. I was a tired first time mom but I was loving every second of it. My baby was very content, unless he was hungry, needed changed or was tired. It took me about 7 weeks to heal and the postpartum part was probably the worst of everything because I was very sore since I had torn.

With our second baby, I was due January 7th 2021. Wednesday January 6th I woke up and started my day with coffee and making breakfast for my toddler. I was also hanging out with my mom, who was staying with us until baby #2 arrived. My fiancé left for work about 8:00 am. At around 9:00 a.m., I started having contractions, but they were mild just like they started with my first baby. I texted my fiancé so he would know. We went about our day and ran some errands, and played with our toddler while I had contractions throughout the day. About 6:00 p.m. we were eating dinner and I could tell my contractions were getting stronger. I wanted to be able to put my toddler to bed before going into the hospital because he decided 4 days before I was due that he was going to crawl out of his crib, so we had to transition him to a toddler bed. He was struggling with this new routine. My mom and I cleaned up the kitchen and I got my toddler ready for bed. My fiancé told me he was going to lay down a bit in case we had to go in soon.

By the time my toddler fell asleep and I walked out of the room, it hit me. My contractions were stronger and I was like, "Oh, no, we need to leave like now!" So I ran in and told my fiancé. I waited for him in the living room, having contractions every 5 minutes. I ran in there to ask him what was taking so long and he had just gotten out of the shower. If looks could kill, he would be dead, but he also didn't realize I was having contractions that close, and was comparing it to my first pregnancy. I was being calm when I came in to tell him we needed to go, so he assumed he could take a quick shower. My mom had put our bags in his truck already. He came out and saw me hunched over in the living room by the door ready to go, and had a shocked look on his face. My mom told me to text her when I get checked in. We got to the hospital at 8:15 p.m. and I was having contractions super close together at this point. They got me checked in and all I was saying was that I wanted the epidural right now. The nurse said, "We need to check you first." They checked me and I was 6 cm! The nurse had me hop up on the bed in between my contractions so they could roll me to the delivery room because at this point I couldn't walk. She then proceeded to tell me that I might be progressing too fast, so I might not be able to have an epidural. This led me into saying, "No, no, no! I want the epidural!"

At this point we were in the delivery room and I was crying/yelling because it hurt. When I was getting on the delivery bed, I was thinking, "I feel his head!" At this point I had a million nurses around me. One had me lay flat as she checked me and called out loud for the doctor. She said, "Sweetie you aren't getting the epidural, your baby is about to come out."

She mumbled it very softly because I think she was scared of what my reaction would be. After she said that, I started cursing. I never curse like that towards anyone or anything, but I was in pain. I swear I couldn't control what I was saying. My fiancé was literally appalled and scared at this point because he had never seen me in pain like that and cursing. I was squeezing my fiancé's hand very tight.

The doctor ran in and she said, "Okay sweetie, I need you to push with this contraction." I did and she said his head was pretty much out, and then she had me push again, and out he came. My fiancé was about to pass out because of my yelling in pain and everything happening so fast. He had to cut the umbilical cord sitting down. My baby was 7 lbs 11.8 oz. We got to the hospital at 8:15 p.m. and I had him at 8:56 p.m. We almost didn't make it! I was in the delivery room for less than 15 minutes after getting checked in.

I apologized to all the nurses for cussing and yelling. I told them I was so embarrassed but I couldn't control what I was saying. They told me that was nothing. When they delivered the placenta it didn't even hurt or anything because I was in such relief holding my baby, and I was glad he was out. So I had an epidural with my first baby and no epidural with my second. My stories are completely different and my babies are completely different.

I Still Had Pain

I've had 4 C-sections. At first I didn't know any different. (I was 20 when I had my first baby.) But when I started to get looks when I said I had a C-section, I began to think I didn't do something right or that I wasn't a "real" mom. I didn't have the pain of pushing a baby out, but I still had pain! It was hard not being able to hold my babies until after I was all stitched up and in the recovery room. My husband held all our children first right next to my head, and I could hold their hands and touch them, but it's hard having to wait.

Your Instincts Take Over

My first childbirth experience was awful. My waters broke spontaneously before labor. With my first, they wouldn't let me do anything but lay on my back. My support wasn't great (inexperienced I think). I ended up having an epidural. Then it got shut off accidentally and I went from 4 cm to 10 cm without it on. Then they turned it on and I couldn't feel anything to push.

23

I almost had to have a C-section, and my doctor was not very patient with the situation.

My second birth was at a different hospital with a different doctor, and it was so much better! I didn't use an epidural and it was such an amazing experience. My third and final pregnancy I ended up having to be induced (after preterm girls and weekly shots, my boy was stubborn). It was mostly a very good experience except I caved and got an epidural, which I've always regretted. I look back at how little I knew about life and parenting when I had my first at 25, compared to my third at 33. I joke that I had no business raising a baby. But your instincts take over and it just becomes natural.

Panic Attack

This was my first child. I went in for my last doctor's appointment before my scheduled induction later in the week. It was on a Monday. I was told I had high blood pressure for the second week in a row and had to go to Labor and Delivery. I went to get checked in and took a COVID test. I got to my room and they started the induction process. I was only dilated 2 cm. They put the balloon in and waited. Later that night they came and told me I had COVID. Once they took the balloon out, I got an epidural. The next day, they broke my water.

Later that night, I found out my epidural had come out so I had to do another one. I was in pain and couldn't tell the end of one contraction from the beginning of another. They gave me medicine that would help with the pain and let me rest. Right after they gave me that, the doctor made the decision to perform a C-section after 20 hours of labor and my baby's heart rate dropping too much. They wheeled me into the room and I fell asleep. I woke up while they were stitching me up. I had a panic attack due to waking up with the blue sheet in front of me and having my mask on. It took them almost an hour due to having a bleeding problem. I was having a panic attack the entire time.

It Wasn't Magical

As a little back story, I had a miscarriage when I was 19 years old. I was 20 weeks along, had just found out I was having a boy, and two nights later I lost him. I had gone to a cheap clinic when it happened. I was so shocked, I never looked at or held him, which I regret to this day. We never found out the true cause of his death. Fast forward to 2019 when I found out I was pregnant with my daughter. I was put on high risk and watched closely throughout the pregnancy because of my history and career as a first responder.

The whole pregnancy I wasn't able to enjoy for many reasons. One was that everyone else seemed to have their own thoughts and opinions about what I should and shouldn't do. I was listening to what my OB and perinatal were telling me. People always wanted to know why they were suggesting me to do certain things and disagreed with them. I was shamed for it and told that I wasn't taking care of my baby the right way. I didn't want to get into details with them as to why I was high risk, which seemed to frustrate them more. They all acted like it was their baby and wanted to tell me what to do, which made the whole experience depressing.

My body had a rough time. My perinatal, OB, and I came up with a plan for birth. We would have NICU on standby and have extra blood for myself and a few other items just in case anything were to happen out of the ordinary. I also had placenta previa up until 34 weeks when they found the placenta had moved just enough for me to be cleared for natural birth. I was super excited for that news. At week 36 I was 1 cm dilated but nothing enough was happening for them to hospitalize me, which I was fine with. When week 38 came along I was still at 1 cm and my OB started to push inducing me early, but I was stubborn. I thought, "Hey, I can prove to everyone that I can make it to 40 weeks." I didn't want to have my baby before or on my birthday. My doctor said at any time I wanted to get the show on the road, or if my water broke, she would be happy to help along.

We decided to induce 3 days later on a Saturday. My doctor wanted me to go sooner, but my birthday was that Friday. I didn't want her on that day for personal reasons. I was up, dressed, packed, and ready to go by 6:00 a.m. on my induction day. We had to be at the hospital at 7:00 a.m. They had to put a balloon inside to help my body dilate because my body was still stuck at 1 cm that morning. They started the process, and everything was ready to go and started by 8:00 a.m.

I loved the RNs I had. One was in training and the other was my main nurse. They offered foot massages and shoulder rubs... AMAZING! I had also texted my family to let them know the eviction notice had been delivered, along with my close friend and doula, who drove all the way down with tons of goodies. My parents showed up as well and would walk around with me and offer to help out with anything my boyfriend or I needed. At 3:26 p.m. they checked the balloon and it came out, so I was finally dilated at 5 cm. At this time I sent my boyfriend home to do a few things he needed to get done and to eat. My mom and dad had stayed and were walking with me after we got the balloon out. All of the sudden, I thought I peed myself. Talk about a weird feeling as an adult! My dad quickly called for the RN. They rushed over to me to help me back to bed. I instructed my mom to call my boyfriend and let him know that my water broke.

At this time I had contractions on top of each other. They asked if I wanted an epidural now or if I wanted to wait. I said, "I want it now." By the time they were ready to give it to me, my boyfriend walked in. I have never been afraid of needles, but this one made me nervous and the contractions were so bad I was in tears. I didn't want my boyfriend, or anyone, to see me like that. He was so sweet and was in front of me talking me through it. He had me rest my head on his chest as they placed it both times. (The first one fell out and I had to do it all over again.)

It was 4:23 p.m. when my doula showed up. Oddly enough my contractions stopped. It literally felt as though time stopped itself. My boyfriend and I updated everything to my doula, who was kind enough to write down all the times for me. She jumped right in and started to do all her doula duties, which I loved. I couldn't have asked for a better doula or friend. I can't thank her enough for all her support and help throughout all of it.

At 7:00 p.m. I was only 7 cm, which was so annoying to me. I was extremely uncomfortable and the only position I could find, the baby's heart rate would drop. Kids have no idea what pain we are willing to go through for them. We did all kinds of things to help get my body going and my baby to go down. She kept trying to wiggle herself back up. The peanut pillow was definitely my favorite thing to have. At 7:40 p.m. they had to put my 3rd epidural in as it popped out again. By 9:00 p.m. I was finally 10 cm and ready to push and got a 4th epidural as it popped out again. Finally, the wait was over, or so I thought.

After 30 minutes of pushing, I was begging to cut her out and saying that I couldn't do it anymore. Thankfully, they listened to my plan, which said to ignore my request for a C-section unless it was necessary. The RN and resident student were coaching me through the pushing while my boyfriend was also by my side helping. It was 12:06 when we had to labor down and get a new epidural as the baby was pushing into my spine and popped it out again. Thankfully, the 5th time was a charm and this one managed to stay put. I also had to get 3 fans on me and be put on oxygen. I ended up passing out a few times throughout the pushing process.

After hours, which felt like days to me, I finally made it to the crowning part. The RN told me to stop pushing as my OB was getting all her stuff on and getting ready for the end. As weak as I felt, my body was still able to finish the job and was pushing my baby out on its own. The RN kept yelling at me to stop pushing, and with a weak voice I was able to say, "It's not me, I am not pushing." My OB calmly looked at me and said, "You can push all you want, the baby isn't going anywhere yet. Don't worry and just listen to your body." I kept saying, "I'm not pushing," and that's when my baby's heart rate started to drop.

My OB advised me to give a big push to get the head out. I didn't have to push that hard and her head popped out. It was my final push due to her being small enough that the rest of her body came out as well. All of the sudden, I saw a blue baby get put on my stomach, wrapped up, and rushed away. My first thought was that my birth plan said I wanted her cleaned off before holding her. Then I realized she was not only blue but not crying, either. I saw the NICU team slowly walk into the room and then rush to our baby. I kept asking what was going on and why wasn't she crying. My OB calmly kept telling me everything was fine and that they are working on her. Knowing what I do for a living, she knew I was aware of what was truly going on and wasn't shy to tell me everything that was happening.

My OB continued to work on me while I looked at my boyfriend who wasn't sure where to go. I told him to go to our baby and stay with her. The next 'fun' part was getting the placenta out. For me it wasn't that bad because I was in and out of it so it didn't bother me much. I did ask to see it, of course. I remember thinking it looked way bigger than I thought it would be. My OB chimed in and said that it actually was very large. She asked if they could run some tests and I approved it. We later would find out that I had two placentas.

Half an hour had passed and I finally heard the sound every new mom expects and wants to hear right away, that first cry. They had spent 30 minutes deep suctioning and working on her to breathe. I wanted to be the first to hold her, but I was still weak at the time and the OB wasn't done with me just yet. My boyfriend got to hold her first. He brought her over to me right away and laid her next to my face in the bed. I'm not too proud of this moment, but I will be honest with you. My first thought when I saw my baby laying there all wrapped up was, "That's it, that's what she looks like? How is that my child?"

For some reason I had it in my head that when I would meet her for the first time, there would be a magical feeling, and there wasn't. This made me wonder why. It turns out it's 100% normal. When they were finally done with me, I was able to hold my daughter for the first time. They finally moved us to our room, where we would stay for a few more days. My daughter not only was a diva in the womb but had to have her own crazy way coming into the world. She has one of the strongest and most independent teenage attitudes that becomes stronger every day. Even though there are things I wish I could go back and change, I learned a ton from having her, which prepared me for the next one.

My Husband Was My Advocate

Both of my births were natural and unmedicated. My first was beautiful, however, I felt disconnected from the situation; I was in a fog. I struggled with postpartum depression. (Later I believe I hemorrhaged.) My second was intense and I was disappointed in my midwife's care and what she was pushing. My husband was my advocate. Recovery was great. I had tons of energy and felt awesome. I felt so much relief and love.

Delivery Was Rough

Afterwards I was shocked and so happy that my babies were here and healthy since my delivery was so rough. All three of my babies were in different incubators. We didn't know who to go to first, so we just stood back where we could see all three in complete awe of how beautiful and healthy they were. I had an absolutely amazing OB/GYN who happened to be walking down the hall when I went into the ER. When the nurses weren't listening to me that I really was in labor and that there was a problem, he stepped in and told them all to, "Move it now." I was rushed right in to get checked out and right into an emergency C-section. Unfortunately, I was put under, and because of problems during the delivery and reactions to anesthetics, I didn't wake up until 8 hours after my kids were born. My poor husband was left in the waiting room, not knowing what was going on.

A Selfless Act

I had always been open to the idea of adoption. My husband wasn't as much. We tried to conceive for about three years and were never able to be pregnant. We started some fertility treatments. We did three rounds of IUI but decided that IVF was not something we wanted to do. At first I wasn't worried about it and just kind of had an "if it happens, it happens" attitude.

28

But when we started trying medical intervention, I was miserable. They had me on hormones that made me not feel like myself. I was angry and emotional.

Eventually my husband came around to the idea of adoption and we started that process. We were blessed to have a short adoption process. We started in February of 2018. We matched with our son's birth mother in April and he was born in August. We were so excited! We started planning and, of course, shopping right away. We did keep it kind of quiet due to the risk of failed adoption, but we told our family, close friends, and coworkers. I think my husband and I both felt bonded with our son right away. They told us that in adoption the bonding process is different because the baby isn't with you for nine months in the womb, so they recommended that we be the only caretakers when we came home. If our son was content, we would let others hold him. But if he was upset, one of us had him. We did all the feedings, diaper changes, baths, bedtime, etc. To be honest, we are still like that, I think, just because we are so used to it from birth.

I just think people need to understand that adoption really is a selfless act on the part of the birth mother. She loved her baby enough to find a family that could give him the life she couldn't. It's not about giving your baby up, it's about wanting more for him. Also, whenever someone places a baby in your arms, they become yours. We feel extremely blessed to have been able to experience the beauty and selflessness of adoption.

Healthy Mom, Healthy Baby Is Not All That Matters

One year ago I tried everything under the sun to induce labor: cleaning, vacuuming, walking, shopping, spicy food, red wine, sex, and bouncing on a ball. And one, or all of them, worked, as I went into labor that night.

I went into my first baby's birth with a bucket full of expectations and preferences and what I thought was the perfect plan. I was going to have this swift, dreamy, unmedicated labor and delivery. And it was going to be perfect. Ultimately we got a perfect baby girl, but her birth? It was absolutely unpredictable. I saw our midwife on Wednesday for my 40 (+1 day) week appointment. She checked me and said I was nearly 4 cm dilated and 70% effaced. After hearing that, I was like, "Woo! labor is going to go so fast!" After all, the first 5 cm take the longest, and I'd done most of that work beforehand.

After waiting what felt like three more years, I woke up with contractions Friday night at 11:45 p.m. After laying in bed through two, trying to decide if they were contractions or not, I got out of bed. At this point, they were between 5-6 minutes apart and 45 seconds long. Immediately, I was feeling the contractions not only in my uterus, but also in my back and thighs. I had to rock through them either on the ball or standing.

We ended up making the decision to go to the hospital around 5:00 a.m. because we had about a half hour drive and I did not want to make that drive with my contractions any closer together. I got to the hospital after hours of contracting, and my midwife told me I was 4 cm and 90% effaced. She could see the defeat in my eyes. I couldn't believe I wasn't any further along! So, it was time to settle in for a long day.

Our doula joined us around 9:00 a.m. and got me to work walking the halls. We tried everything imaginable to get the labor out of my back: walking, position changing, the ball, the tub... EVERYTHING. And nothing brought me relief other than trusty rice packs and a heck of a ton of pressure on my lower back. Later in the afternoon I was checked again and had only progressed to 6 cm. SIX CENTIMETERS! I was discouraged that I hadn't progressed further and faster. This is not what I expected.

At this point, we decided to have my water broken to see if it would speed up labor. So, my midwife broke my water and discovered our sweet girl had passed some meconium. At four days overdue, it wasn't surprising. She was ready to make her debut. Unfortunately, this meant that the NICU team would have to be present for her birth to assess her and make sure she was healthy. Ugh. Disappointment.

The hour after getting my water broken was really a blur. I felt like I was dying. With each and every contraction, I struggled more to stay on top of them and keep my cool. The back and thigh labor I was experiencing was straight from satan himself, and I wouldn't wish that pain on anyone. I am convinced that any woman who has had this kind of labor is a special kind of superwoman. I got to the point where I was suffering through contractions and not just struggling to cope. So I begged for relief, knowing that I would not have this baby without an epidural.

My midwife and doula had the same conversation with me that I've had with a number of clients who had wanted to labor and deliver unmedicated. My body was not progressing fast enough and I needed the help to relax and help my cervix get complete. I hadn't lost or failed. I got the epidural around 4:00 p.m., having progressed 7 cm after 16 hours of labor. Finally, relief from the unimaginable back labor. I still had quite the range of motion with the epidural, allowing me to help my husband, doula, and nurse move me into different positions. For a few hours I switched between laboring on my sides and hands and knees.

At 8:00 p.m., my body was finally complete and I was ready to push. Thanks to the perfect epidural, I was able to push on my sides and hands and knees. I loved being able to feel when I was having a contraction and still having the ability to push in a number of positions. I pushed and I pushed and I pushed. My midwife could tell that my baby was a little wonky (asynclitic) in the birth canal and needed to be adjusted. She called in an OB, who was able to turn her head. After the OB turned her, he gave me more time to push, but she still wasn't coming. He told me he thought she was having a difficult time coming under my pelvic bone and thought that an episiotomy would help her make her way out.

This is not what I wanted! I knew the risks. Through hysterical tears I said, "NO!" to everyone in the room, but I finally consented because this baby wasn't going to be born otherwise. After demanding more pain medication, because up until this point I could feel everything with every push (pressure, contractions coming on, and a wicked hemorrhoid), he gave me an episiotomy. And after about three contractions, she was born at 10:50 p.m., with nearly three hours of pushing.

As soon as she came out, my husband cut her cord and she was taken over to the other side of the room to be assessed by the NICU team. There was no delayed cord clamping. My husband wasn't able to help catch her. She wasn't placed right on my chest. I cried. A lot. I cried because I was happy she had finally arrived. I cried because nothing went the way I wanted it to go. Our incredible doula just cradled my head, while my husband went with our daughter to be assessed. He immediately ran over and told me just how beautiful she was. Thankfully, once she was given the okay, my husband was able to carry her over and put her on my chest. She was beautiful. And perfect. And she had hair! She was so alert. I couldn't believe she was ours.

After 23 hours, and the hardest day of my life, our daughter was born, and she was healthy and beautiful. The day went nothing like I had expected, but she was here! And I was healthy and well. To some extent I'm still disappointed that so many things didn't go according to "plan," but I don't regret any consent I gave or interventions I okayed, because we're both healthy. It was like God gave me this "not according to plan" birth story for my first child to teach me that in no way is the experience that I wanted and lost out on worth more than her life and mine.

A little word on, "Healthy mom, healthy baby, that's all that matters." Yes. This does matter THE MOST. But it's not ALL that matters. A mother's experience matters as well. While I understand this sentiment and why people say it, let's think before we say it because the last thing I want to do is discount or devalue a mother's experience during the birth of her child.

According To Plan

I woke up at 5:30 a.m. and quickly went from, "I think I may be leaking amniotic fluid," to "I'm leaking. We're having a baby today." We quickly packed our bags, tossed the car seat in the car, showered, and my mom came over. My oldest daughter woke up early, like she knew what was going on. We gave her kisses and were out the door by 7:00 a.m. I had been feeling aches in my back through packing and the drive over, but once we were in L&D, things pretty much stopped. My midwife came in to check on me, and I was already 3 cm. We got an IV started, and I hopped onto the ball around 9:30 a.m. to do some nipple stimulation to help kick labor into gear, all while texting a friend about how I couldn't believe I was having my baby and sending her selfies. Contractions soon came back in regularity and strength.

Once we kick-started labor without Pitocin, my midwife got me up and walking the halls. At this point, contractions were growing in intensity and I was squatting during some of them, and walking through a few, but having one each lap. We went back to the room around 11:00 a.m. and I was 5 cm. I hopped into the tub and we texted our photographer to arrive at noon since things were speeding up. At this point, things got real. Contractions were strong and consistent. I'm so thankful for our midwife's strong hands and both she and my husband's encouraging words on how well I was coping and to keep going. They both used a lot of touch for pain relief, while encouraging me to breathe and moan through them. My midwife checked me again and I was 8 cm at 11:39 a.m. My husband texted the photographer to HURRY and I got out of the tub. Everything past this is a mixture of being a blur but also unforgettable. Our photographer showed up while I was transitioning and nearly clawing my husband's shirt off coping with the intensity. Once they were able to coax me onto the bed and in the hands and knees position, my midwife checked me again and it was time to push at 12:07 p.m.

After only about ten minutes of pushing, and a lot of yelling at my midwife, our baby was born at 12:20 p.m. I delivered her on my hands and knees, and after flipping over, she was brought right to my chest. Such joy. Such relief. Such shock. So many feelings. I did it! Thanks to all the support, I birthed my baby girl without pain medication or any interventions -- a completely different experience from my first labor and delivery. I still can't quite believe it. I can't believe how it felt. I can't believe how fast it went and how much I remember. Thankfully, despite being early, we didn't have any baby drama and were able to enjoy the sacred hour together, have delayed cord clamping, and even give nursing a go. While we worked with our baby girl on her feeding, as she went to the NICU, I remained so grateful that I was able to give birth exactly according to my birth plan this time around. What an absolutely incredible experience, one I'll surely never forget.

Everything Was Pretty Chill

I went into my suite at 8:30 p.m. to be induced. My friend was with me while I was waiting on mom and dad to make the 15 hour trek to be there. Everything was pretty chill, aside from not being able to get comfortable due to the monitors coming off the baby every time I fell asleep. At 4:25 a.m., my water broke. After that, everything went very quickly.

I went into this all thinking I was going to do a natural birth, having done my research. Going from 3 cm to 8 cm in about 20 minutes had me throwing up and saying otherwise. By around 6:00 a.m., I had an epidural and then my parents arrived from their trip. I saw my OB at 7:00 a.m., and then I took a nice nap before the festivities started. She came back just before 10:00 a.m. and told me it was time and that we were going to have to start pushing before it was too late. After a short 20 minutes, my baby was here at 10:16 a.m. All in all, I'm glad I didn't have a solid plan going in because I also didn't have any disappointments with myself.

She Makes Me Strive to Better Myself

Birth made me feel like Wonder Woman! My baby ended up tearing me from end to end with a level 4 tear. The doctors and nurses wanted to pump me full of pain meds for it, but it didn't hurt, so I refused. They were stunned that it didn't hurt. I was able to create such a wonderful human who is now one of the most polite girls I've ever met. She is also not afraid to stick up for herself and even for others. My daughter is a great friend, and to this day she still makes me strive to better myself for her.

Both Traumatic and Beautiful

I truly do not remember too many people being around me during the birth experience who I felt were very supportive. I definitely had to advocate for myself during the laboring process. An example of this was being diagnosed with preeclampsia. I knew that my blood pressure systolic reading was abnormal, but the nurse kept telling me I was fine. I had to beg for a blood test, which confirmed preeclampsia.

My husband is very supportive but tends to shy away from hospitals and medical intervention. He freezes up a bit. He was next to me the entire time I was pushing to birth our daughter, but I do not remember much of him being there. I hired a doula to be at my birth. I was supposed to have a C-section that morning, and when my baby flipped on her own, the doula that I hired had to leave because she was not planning to be there all day. Another doula came to relieve her, but she did not arrive until late in the evening. Although she was helpful when she did arrive, it was disheartening to have my water broken and labor all afternoon feeling alone.

No one was specifically rude, but I definitely didn't feel heard on many topics. Right after my daughter's birth, I do remember the doctor saying, "I just had to get stern with you at the end." She was referring to my pushing ability and how I needed to get my baby out quickly. That rubbed me the wrong way because it insinuated that I wasn't trying previously, and gave the doctor credit for "coaching," when I felt like I was working as hard as I could.

I do feel that medical personnel are interested in learning other service delivery models, and we need to teach them various ways of birthing babies to allow the mother to be the expert of her body. My birthing experience is unique in that it comes from the perspective of a women's health and specialized pelvic floor occupational therapist. For instance, as I was birthing my daughter, I was explaining to the nurses my breathing techniques and why my methods were different from what they were instructing me to do. They were very curious and supportive of this. The most empowering part was having choices because I never stopped educating myself. I even switched providers at 36 weeks to have my voice be heard and feel like I was part of the decision making process. Regardless of the type of birth (vaginal or cesarean) I felt at peace and centered. I felt proud of my body and the journey that my baby and I had gone on. No one could take that from us.

One's birthing experience does not have to fit neatly into a definable box. Birth, pregnancy, labor and delivery can all be both traumatic and beautiful. The two are not mutually exclusive. It is OK to have to heal from something, even when you consider the experience a positive one.

VBAC Stories

VBAC stands for vaginal birth after cesarean. Nearly 40% of hospitals in the United States still have some form of VBAC ban, which makes repeat cesareans mandatory. VBAC moms often face many obstacles finding a supportive provider, even though research says it's safe. If you were ever told, "Once a C-section, always a C-section," I encourage you to research your options. There are so many possibilities when it comes to childbirth.

My Doctor Was Wrong

I feel like my VBACs were the most powerful experiences of my life. I went from a woman who didn't challenge the programming in place that created beliefs about birth, to a strong fearless mother who will know all of her options before making any important decision that impacts her family. My gut told me that my doctor was wrong when she said I'd always have to have a C-section because my pelvis was too small. I started exploring other options and found VBAC, specifically VBAC at home.

Do not neglect preparing mentally for birth. We focus a lot on diet and preparing our body, but we forget about the emotional and mental work that needs to be done. You have every right to try to birth a baby the way you were designed! Sometimes we just have to uncover the power that is within us.

It Would Be a Fight

I felt robbed when I had a C-section. I felt angry that nobody would attend a vaginal breech birth. I had a decent cesarean as far as those go. I was treated with respect and I wasn't tied down. We were able to take photos and a video of it, but I was not allowed to do skin to skin in the OR. I also was not allowed to have her with me in recovery. I didn't have any immediate direct complications, but it made breastfeeding harder and I had postpartum depression.

I knew the impact my cesarean would have on my future childbearing and birth options. My mom had a VBAC in the 1980's, so I knew it was an option, but I also knew it would be a fight. I have had two VBACs since my first was born. One was at home and the other at the hospital. Thirteen years later, I feel differently about my C-section. I did the best I could do with the circumstances and resources I had at the time. I know my body even better now, and I have precipitous labors. In the future I would go wherever I need to go to at least attempt a breech VBAC.

I Trust My Body

Having a VBAC has changed my outlook on birth. It has changed the way I trust my body and rely on the process of birth. I wanted, and needed, to heal from my traumatic cesarean with my first son. My idea of birth was based around fear after that traumatic experience. My water broke at 37 weeks, 4 days. After laboring for 11 hours, I was stalled at 9.5 cm for 2 hours before my OB called for a C-section. My baby was never in distress. My body was not given the chance to do what it was made to do. I put all of my trust in the OB, instead of trusting my body.

My boyfriend and I didn't know what to expect with it being our first, so we just went along with what the OB said. I was never asked before anything was done. I felt more pain than I should've during my C-section. While my arms were strapped down, I was crying. The anesthesiologist was scrolling through Facebook, reminding me to be still, while not taking his eyes off of the screen. When my baby was pulled from me, I didn't get to see him or hold him until he'd been poked and prodded and weighed.

I was extremely happy my baby was finally here, and I trusted the OB that my body just couldn't birth a baby vaginally. It wasn't until I really reflected on my birth experience that I decided I would trust my body and try for a VBAC with my second baby. I found out I was pregnant with baby number two in February 2019. That's when my search began for the birthing team I wanted to make my VBAC happen.

I did lots of research into different OBs, hospitals and midwives. I joined the ICAN group on Facebook, and that's where I learned about the Midwives at UNMC and their wonderful VBAC rates. After my first appointment, I was so thrilled and excited for the birth of my second. I also began my search for a doula, also recommended by the ICAN group for VBAC mamas. That's when I found one. Her birth story of her first baby made me feel like I had someone on my team that understood my trauma, and her birth of her second baby completely inspired me! My team was complete, and I spent the following months prepping my mind and telling myself and everyone that asked that I was going to have a VBAC. I didn't even let myself think of the "what ifs".

My son's story starts about 3 weeks before he actually came into this world. I was a little over 34 weeks when the contractions started about 4-7 minutes apart for most of the day. I was in touch with my doula, and we both thought it was a good idea that I go into L&D and be monitored. When I arrived, one of the midwives asked if it was OK if she checked to see if I was dilated. I was at 1 cm & 50% effaced. She decided they'd continue to monitor for an hour. I could tell the contractions were getting closer together, and I called her back in the room.

She was in the room, about to send me home and tell me to rest and hydrate, when my contractions dropped to 3 minutes apart. She then asked if she could perform another cervical check. I agreed and I was 2 cm & 60 % effaced. I was admitted for the next 3 days. While I was there, I was given steroids to mature my baby's lungs. I never progressed anymore in those 3 days. Baby decided he wasn't ready, and ultimately that was the best thing that could've happened. We really wanted to avoid NICU time.

The next 3 weeks were full of prodromal labor. I didn't know how I'd possibly make it to 42 weeks if my baby wanted to bake as long as possible. I knew my chances of having a successful VBAC went down if I was induced, so I spent the time taking lots of baths and talking to my baby. It was at my 37 week appointment that the midwives told me that they knew I was becoming miserable with constant contractions, but they weren't causing any cervical change. My baby would come when he was ready, whether it be that night or at 42 weeks. Contractions picked up even more that afternoon. I thought nothing of it because I'd been contracting for 3 weeks. I decided I'd take a bath, watch Netflix, and go to bed early that night. I kept waking up every couple hours just feeling sick to my stomach. Around 12:00 a.m., I decided to go lay in bed.

Around 1:40 a.m. I woke, sat up, and felt a huge pop. I knew my water had broken and the contractions almost immediately got super intense. I called my doula to let her know that my water had broken and I thought maybe it was meconium stained. My boyfriend and I headed to the hospital, and my doula said she'd meet us there. When we got into the delivery room, the midwife and nurse made sure I really was ruptured, and I was. Upon arrival I was 3 cm and almost all the way effaced. After about an hour, I was asked if they could check my cervix for progress, and I was at 6 cm in one hour. After about 2 hours I was struggling with managing my pain and all thoughts of a medication free birth went out the window. Although I would've loved to be able to do it, it didn't happen for me at this birth. The epidural gave me that break I needed to pick myself back up and continue to bring my baby into the world. Little did I know once I progressed to 7 cm I would stall for 5 hours. Along with stalling, my epidural was causing a whole other set of issues, including horrible neck spasms, fever, and super high heart rate in myself. This all persisted until my baby was born.

My boyfriend and my doula were constantly reminding me how strong I was and that I actually could do it when I felt like giving up. My baby was not in the most ideal position, and I was stalling because of that. My doula helped me into different positions to get my baby's head out of the wonky position, and it worked! Baby was where he needed to be now and I began dilating again. 18 hours in, I started feeling immense pressure. The midwife checked me again and I was 9 cm with a cervical lip. At this point I truly don't believe my epidural was even functioning correctly because I felt everything, and I'm so glad I was able to. My baby's heart rate started getting a little higher, indicating that he was getting tired. My midwife sat down on the bed next to me and let me know what was going on and told me all of my options. She said we could wait and give our baby a little more time to try and come, or that I could choose to have a C-section. I was absolutely determined to have my VBAC. I knew our baby would come if I gave him a little more time. The urge to push was getting more and more intense. I just knew I had to be at 10 cm by this point, and I was! My instinct was not to push laying on my back and instead I used the squatting bar. My legs were numb from the epidural, so I honestly don't know how I pulled this off. With each push, I felt less and less pain, and it was almost comforting. I didn't need to be coached; my body knew what to do and I was in my zone. In under 25 minutes of pushing, my baby was finally here and he was put right on my chest. I felt an instant sense of relief and excitement that I did it.

I gave birth vaginally even after being told I wouldn't be able to after my first birth. I had no tearing whatsoever. I contribute that to not being on my back while pushing the whole time. My baby latched beautifully the first time, something that I struggled with my first baby. After the first couple hours, my baby was weighed and measured. He was the exact weight as my first, and his head was even bigger than my first. I not only was successful at birthing him vaginally, this proved to me that I could've also birthed my first if given the time for my body to do what it's made to do.

Indescribable

When I found out my second baby was breech, I immediately asked the midwife about options for providers in the hospital system who perform vaginal breech births. She gave me the name of an OB who would do it. I called the same day to see if I could get in (at 32 weeks), just in case my baby didn't flip and an ECV didn't work. This helped me to feel empowered, like the decision was up to me and not a provider who would automatically do a C-section. I ended up having a breech VBAC, and it was the hardest thing I've ever done. It was indescribable, empowering and affirming.

Having a provider experienced in vaginal breech birth was huge for me. She had criteria that I had to meet in order to do it. I trusted that my baby would arrive safely, regardless of how he was born. I was able to release my fears and trust her the whole way.

It Was Amazing

I had two vaginal births, then a C-section for my 28 week premature baby due to him being breech. 15 months later, I had a successful VBAC. I went into labor on my own at 40 weeks. My doctor would have let me go 42 weeks before induction. I was patient and let my body do what it was meant to do. When I started pushing, my contractions stopped. My doctor let my body push the baby out instead of forcing my baby out, which would have strained both of us. It was amazing to just sit and let it all happen on its own.

Follow Your Instincts

With my first cesarean, I was relieved. My baby was breech and I did not want an EVC. I was relieved to have a set date because my husband wasn't going to miss the birth. He was military, overseas, and on a 15 day leave window (including travel) for the birth. We had struggled with infertility for years prior, and I did not want him to miss our child's birth.

With our second baby, though, I was frustrated. I was labeled a "failure to progress TOLAC." I felt like the moment that I entered the hospital, the odds were stacked against me. The hospital's policy at that time was that I had to labor in bed. With our third child, I was heartbroken. I had planned a VBA2C from the beginning. At 36 weeks, both VBAC doctors left the practice. The other doctors were only pro repeat C-section. I was not familiar with the birth community where I delivered my third, so I felt my options were limited. I then opted for a "gentle family centered caesarean."

I am proud of my VBA3C because I educated and advocated for myself. I fought hard for it! I delivered during the pandemic, with an unsupportive provider. Originally, my care was with a supportive midwife. We planned a home birth. I was receiving prenatal co-care with a supportive OB just in case. We ended up in a hospital transfer due to complications while the supportive provider was still there. Shift change gave me an unsupportive provider, and then I had to fight for it. My feelings about my VBA3C are mixed though, because I ended up with some major birth trauma from the delivering provider and hospital. My husband is a trucker now, which means lots of solo parenting for me. He was only going to have 1 ½ weeks off after my baby's birth. My other three children were 8 and under. I needed a shorter recovery time. Plus, I just did not want to be cut open again.

When the unsupportive provider said that I would be having a repeat C-section, I refused. Neither mine nor my baby's health were at risk. He only wanted to do a repeat because he did not feel comfortable with the liability of a VBA3C. I had an amazing nurse who advocated strongly for me, too. She got both the nurse manager and patient advocacy involved to fight for my rights as a patient. My advice to others seeking a VBAC would be to educate and advocate for yourself. Follow your instincts. Surround yourself with supportive people and providers. Ignore the naysayers.

It Was Best for Us

My VBAC was empowering and it was exciting to feel like I could do it. It has made me a bigger fighter and advocate for myself. With my cesarean, I was sad. I felt like the system failed me (it did), and I was motivated to never have one again unless absolutely necessary. I wanted a VBAC because my C-section was a joke. It was not not necessary and I knew I could do it the right way. I wanted all of the benefits for my baby of going through labor and through the vagina. I just knew it was what was best for me and my baby. I held on to that conviction.

I ended up tearing really badly, 3rd degree, with internal tears as well. The recovery for me was worse than my cesarean. I never thought I'd say that, but now I know what my goal for the next baby will be. I don't regret it for one minute. I am still happy I did it and plan to do a second HBAC. It was the way God intended it to be. During my HBAC I was focused on my baby and not worried at all about all the "statistics" they use to deter you from trying. It was so natural and it was birth as it was meant to be. My advice is to surround yourself with people who support you. If someone doesn't, it's okay that they don't understand. You don't need everyone to be on board, but definitely find your team you can trust.

It Didn't Have to Be Stressful

After we found out our baby was breech, they booked me for a C-section the next day. I was 40 weeks + 1 day at the time. Apparently the hospital's only option was repeated C-section, as I was a VBAC candidate with post-date breech presentation. I was absolutely devastated. I'd worked so hard mentally and emotionally for a VBAC, and I felt like it had been ripped from me. My hospital didn't support breech VBAC. My baby did, in fact, turn head down at the last minute. I went into the booked C-section the next day. They told me they had to do a last minute scan. My options were to continue with the C-section, be induced, or go home. With all my strength I chose to go home. I went home with the fear he would flip back as I was 40 weeks+2 days at that time. I went into labor that afternoon and birthed my baby the next day. The experience didn't have to be that stressful before the birth of my baby, but it was. Nothing about my care was women-centered. The lack of trust they have in women's bodies is baffling.

My Body Is Capable

Cesareans are a blessing to have when necessary, but they are massively overused. They are normalized, when they should be considered a rare occurrence. My first VBAC was very healing for me. With my first baby, which turned into a C-section, it was a very traumatic experience. It was bad enough that it left me not ever wanting anymore kids. When I was planning my VBAC I went into it fully trusting my body and not allowing a single person to interfere with that. If someone didn't support me, I had no room for them in my birth space, physically or emotionally. Having my son at home as a VBAC was everything I needed to validate what I already knew -- my body is capable and strong.

With my second VBAC I was able to just fully give myself to my birth experience with no hesitation or need to lean on anyone for support. I spent it very inner focused. I didn't need anyone to remind me to relax, open up and breathe. I knew my body could do it. I did not want to go through another experience of going to the ER, being strapped down, and separated from my new baby for hours and missing everything while they did a bath and everything else they wanted to.

My advice is to trust yourself, your body, your inner voice and your instincts. It's okay to stand up and say this is what is going to happen. Talk through any fears with someone who supports a VBAC (supports, not tolerates, there is a huge difference). Don't be afraid to fire a provider if they don't fully support your choice. They work for you; you can tell them to take a hike and find a provider who does support you.

Changed My Life

My first two cesareans were okay, but my third gave me anxiety. With my fourth baby, I didn't consent to surgery unless I needed it. Having a VBAC changed my whole life, the whole of who I am.

Worth Investing the Best Support

With my cesarean, I felt very detached from the experience. The whole thing felt like it was happening to me, as opposed to me being a part of the experience. I hated that I was so out of it from anesthesia that I didn't remember hearing my baby cry when he was born. I also didn't like the idea that I carried this baby for 9 months to get to be maybe the 5th person to hold my baby. Unfortunately (fortunately?), it was planned, due to breech position, but I had spontaneous labor before the scheduled cesarean. I didn't labor long -- though I did get to experience what it was like, and it did happen spontaneously.

The operation itself went "textbook," but 8 hours later I passed out due to postpartum hemorrhage. My body was also forming a ton of clots that required a manual D&C at the bedside, which was excruciating, despite my tap block and narcotic pain medicine. As it turned out, I continued to hemorrhage for 3 weeks postpartum, due to undiagnosed "uterine atony," which culminated in me passing a clot the size of a softball. I went back to the OB, and with a 24 hour prescription for Methergine, it quickly resolved. Because of my complications that happened postpartum, not actually in the OR, my whole birth experience felt very traumatic, beyond just feeling detached from the OR. I also clearly don't respond well to anesthesia of any kind because apparently most moms post-op spend roughly an hour in recovery, just long enough for the spinal to wear off so they can help transfer beds, and it took 3 hours for me. The thought of not regaining my legs back (perhaps, somewhat unrealistic), and knowing for most women it wears off within an hour, was scary.

Simply put, my first birth experience was traumatic to me, and I just couldn't SIGN UP for another experience like that. Because my first was traumatic, in my mind, even though I know it's not black and white like this, having a C-section = having a traumatic experience. Scheduling a repeat cesarean felt like promising to repeat my first experience, and I couldn't just sign up for that. If something happened and it resulted in that, OK, but to electively enter into it felt incomprehensible.

My first provider used a lot of the scare tactics related to uterine rupture and hysterectomy on me, but we always said we wanted 3-4 kids, and I did not want 3-4 kids badly enough to be cut open that many times. If my second birth experience was anywhere near as traumatic as my first, I couldn't mentally and emotionally enter into a third pregnancy anyway, so I'd have been done at two anyhow. So I guess my logic also was, "Well, if I have a uterine rupture that ends up being catastrophic and results in a hysterectomy... I was gonna end up being done after two babies anyway (if I had a second cesarean) because I wasn't going to sign up for a third anyhow."

There were also just so many things I didn't like about the cesarean, OR and that experience. I was determined to just have a different experience. I felt like my husband got to experience my cesarean birth, not me. Even though I was awake, I was really in and out, wanting to fall asleep and just barely coherent. I don't even remember hearing my baby cry, and that felt devastating to me. I didn't like that I wasn't a part of the experience, that it just happened to me. I was told, "You'll feel some tugging and pulling," but not, "and we're pulling the baby out!" I didn't even know when he was born. The fact that they carry on their own random conversation as if you're not lying there awake, cut open on a table, as if you're not there, feels weird. I get this is routine for them, but this should be an intimate experience for me, and they don't treat it, or you, like that in an OR.

I remember feeling like I was going to vomit, and being slightly terrified I'd choke on it and die because how else would I use my stomach muscles to heave while I'm cut open?! Thankfully, I said that, and the anesthesiologist was able to push something to make it go away. I remember being in recovery and them talking about how it usually takes about 1 hour for the spinal to wear off and that I was approaching the 3 hour mark. I started to become fearful that I may never get the feeling back in my legs, when I'd have otherwise opted for a natural childbirth (without an epidural), because I don't like not being in control of my body. It was more than my postpartum hemorrhage. It was more than the incredibly impersonal nature of an OR delivery, more than feeling detached and having it all happening to me, and more than a C-Section recovery/healing from a MAJOR abdominal surgery. With all of it combined, I couldn't do it again electively. The only way I was going into the OR again was if it was a life and death situation.

My water broke at 34 weeks and 5 days. We waited out 17 hours for labor to start, but it did not, so we consented to Pitocin. I was also GBS+ and my baby was now going to be premature. I consented to antibiotics in labor hoping it would buy us some time and prevent infection. Thankfully, it seemed to do just that. 30 hours on Pitocin later, at 35 weeks, our baby came via VBAC, at 46.5 hours ROM (rupture of membranes). A VBAC tolerant provider would have likely cut me off at 24 hours ROM, but my provider did not. Neither me, nor my baby had any signs of infection, and we were both stable, so there was no need to resort to surgery just due to a timeline. I also stalled at 6 cm for seven hours. ACOG (American College of Obstetricians and Gynecologists) states that, "failure to progress" is "stalling at 6 cm for six hours or more," which happened to me. If my provider was practicing in accordance with ACOG and evidence based birth guidelines (which would have been respectable because many OBs sadly are not), he could have sent me to surgery because I "qualified," but he didn't. He was okay with time. Interestingly enough for about the last 10 hours of my labor, I was 100% effaced and my baby was at station +2. When my OB came in and checked me, I was still at 6 cm for seven hours at that point with a pliable cervix. He was able to manually dilate me the rest of the way to help my baby come successfully via VBAC and not resort to surgery. THAT is what a pro-VBAC doctor does. They help you achieve the birth experience you desire without their own desire, agenda, or convenience.

Having a VBAC was life changing, and I'm not even sure I could count the ways. I guess at the most basic level, it has spurred me on to provide a platform for educating and informing women. It certainly ignited a passion for me in helping women know that they can, and how to, advocate for themselves. A fellow VBAC mom friend and I started a local ICAN chapter in our area when our VBAC babies (born 2 days apart) were about 18 months old. We thought it was the best way to at least provide a platform for women to come and be informed, and supported. I truly feel like the veil has been torn and now I see so clearly. Sadly, what I see is all the injustice in the birth world. OBs aren't practicing in accordance with ACOG (their certifying board) guidelines. They aren't giving women informed consent. They aren't practicing EVIDENCE BASED deliveries or prenatal care. They aren't learning about all things related to perinatal care, from lactation consultants and nursing, and postpartum doulas, to pelvic floor physical therapy, and Webster certified chiropractors.

I can't quite say I feel called to being a doula. It would be challenging for me to support a mom who "concedes" to a cesarean, but it isn't off the table either. I switched at 25 weeks during my 2nd pregnancy to a more pro-VBAC provider, and as a MFM (DO, not an MD) male, he acted more like a midwife than the actual midwives did at the practice I was previously at. That was eye opening that females aren't a better OB, nor can we make the generalization that "midwives are better than OBs." He also provided such a high level of care and concern (at one point with my first provider, I felt I had to sacrifice empathy for "care"), that it shifted my approach to what I look for out of ALL of my medical providers: dentist, pediatrician, primary care, etc.

My advice to anyone planning a VBAC: surround yourself with supportive people. If someone's not supportive, share as little as possible, don't engage in birth related conversation with them, or just avoid them/the topic altogether. Educate, educate, educate. Don't assume your provider's recommendations are evidence based, or "what's best" for you. Sadly, I've found that most aren't. Take a birth class you have to pay for that's not in the hospital. Get a doula. Invest as much into this birth experience (time and financially) and prepare your body for delivery as you would ANY other goal you have in life. There are very few life events as significant as the birth experience of your child. It's worth investing in the best support: a good prenatal massage therapist, a Webster certified Chiropractor and more. Don't be afraid to switch providers. You are paying them for a service, just the same you would at a restaurant. If the service was poor or the food wasn't good, you wouldn't hesitate to not go back. You aren't married to your provider and no amount of their "niceness" will help you achieve your birth experience. If how they practice doesn't scream pro-VBAC, detach yourself from the emotional tie to the provider, and consider the facts. Also, don't be afraid to drive farther for a more supportive provider. You're more likely to wonder, "What if I had just given in to the drive," If you don't get that VBAC.

He Is Perfect

My first son wouldn't descend after 24 hours. His heart rate started to drop, and we were rushed into a C-section. It was really hard because I had planned for a natural birth and had no clue about C-sections. I hadn't even thought of it as a possibility. We spent a week in the NICU due to infection. He had to be transferred before I could hold him, which was the hardest part. I followed 18 hours after my C-section. It was super hard to not have the care from the hospital anymore.

With my second son, my pregnancy was super normal. My boys are 20 months apart, and although I wanted to give birth at a birth center instead of a hospital, it was "too risky." I went into labor with my second son and after 6 hours went into the hospital. The nurse was thinking I'd be going back home because I was so calm during contractions, but I was at 5-6 cm. I worked through them for the next 20 hours and started to use nitrous. They just left me alone for the most part because I was progressing, just slowly.

At about 30 hours and 9 cm, I got the epidural. I was so tired and just needed to rest. Baby was still super high and they thought I had a little while to go. After a couple hours my contractions slowed, so they gave me very low Pitocin. At 35 hours, my epidural ran out and I was in intense pain. They started it back up but it never totally went away. I started to push and was able to give birth to my son vaginally after 15-20 minutes. He came really fast, but needed CPAP right away, so I only held him for a second.

I kept experiencing really intense pain in my upper abdomen. I have a super high pain tolerance and thought I had demonstrated this throughout my labor, but the nurses still brushed me off when I tried to tell them. They thought it was just contractions after birth, even when I told them it was a constant pain. I asked for pain medication to cope because I couldn't even manage to hold my son, and they said I would have to have an ultrasound first.

I got an ultrasound, which showed fluid in my abdomen, and then I was taken for a CT scan. I could barely move but had to get on and off the hard plastic board and lay still for the scan, which was excruciating. During the scan, they found that my uterus had ruptured and they rushed me into surgery. It was about 2 hours after birth. They were able to repair my uterus and remove the blood in my abdomen. I had to have a large blood transfusion because I had lost so much but I felt so much better afterwards. I was able to room in with my son, and we spent 5 days in the hospital being cared for and successfully breastfeeding. He is perfect in every way, just like his older brother.

All Kinds of Anxiety

I felt my C-section was necessary, but I also felt cheated. I didn't get to hold my son until a few hours after he was born, and I feel robbed of those first hours. Having a VBAC helped me feel empowered to advocate for myself in making healthcare decisions for me and for my child. It also gave me a sense of relief that I could have a baby "normally" and my body was not somehow broken. My husband and I want a large family. I was scared of the increased risk of placenta accreta with repeated C-sections. I knew finding a supportive provider would be astronomically harder with repeated C-sections, and I wanted the easier recovery with vaginal birth so I could be fully present for my baby and my family.

I got to experience navigating the healthcare system during a pandemic, arguing with doctors who were not following evidence based care and switching practices twice. I also experienced all kinds of anxiety around whether I was being foolish to argue with the doctors (although my research told me otherwise), additional risk factors of gestational diabetes, pregnancy at maternal age of 35, gestational hypertension, and anxiety about baby's position since my firstborn was breech. I eventually switched to a freestanding birth center and had my daughter exactly on her due date. After two days of off-on labor that I thought wasn't doing anything, my water broke and my contractions reached 3-5 minutes apart. My husband and I headed to the birth center, which was 30 minutes away. My contractions never got much closer, but I walked in the door of the birth center and she was born 20 minutes later! I got to deliver on my hands and knees, which was what I wanted, and I had no tearing. Baby was perfect and I was home and up walking around later that day.

Healing and Empowering

When I had my cesarean, I felt thankful because it brought my baby boy into the world. But I also held a lot of resentment toward my body for not doing the "right" thing. My first child's birth felt out of my control in so many ways I can't even begin to list. I wanted some kind of control. Some kind of power. To feel like my body was mine again and it was capable and strong.

My VBAC was so healing and empowering. I made my mind up that was what I was going to do, and I did everything in my power to avoid another cesarean. I powered through multiple false alarms and 36 hours of contractions to get there.

Just a few things: If the nurse tells you not to go to the bathroom because you could have the baby on the toilet, they are probably right. A good nurse will advocate for you and cheer you on, while a bad one will roll their eyes when they say it's your last chance for an epidural and you refuse it. I always thought it would be so weird to watch myself give birth in a mirror, but it was actually helpful and encouraging.

CBAC Stories

CBAC stands for cesarean birth after cesarean. It sounds repetitive, but this is a term that is specifically reserved for mothers who have a repeat cesarean after attempting a VBAC. When I had my second cesarean, I found that there was a whole demographic of people who felt similar to me. We planned and prepared so hard for a VBAC that didn't happen. In some ways it seems that we put VBAC moms on a pedestal. We see their stories as inspiring and may even think, "She faced all of these obstacles; she's a hero!" I want to remind you that you also worked hard for a VBAC (maybe even harder). Your stories are inspiring and valid. You're heroes, too.

Birth Is Complicated

Having a CBAC was devastating, but also more empowering than my first birth because I was treated with the dignity and respect lacking in my first birth. I know that I did all that I could and loved my baby enough to care so much about their birth. Birth is beautiful no matter how it turns out. Having a CBAC is not due to doing something wrong. Many people attribute the "success or failure" of a VBAC to their own efforts. Either they did everything to prepare, or they didn't do enough, but in reality, birth is complicated and there is some luck involved. Those who have VBACs and those who have CBACs would all do well to remember that.

It Changed Me Forever

My first was a planned home birth. We transferred to the hospital during the pushing stage because my baby wasn't descending. I felt supported during the whole experience, but it was the comments after the birth from insensitive people that left me feeling lacking. The people I thought would show up (mom and mother-in-law) kept cancelling. I was alone because my husband had to go back to work 5 days postpartum. I found myself silently screaming in the shower. Hopelessness. Rage. Hurt. There was physical pain like I had never experienced.

My second pregnancy I planned a VBAC with a midwife. I had an induction with foley and Pitocin at 41 weeks due to low amniotic fluid and a big baby estimate. The induction went well, and I felt really supported, but my baby stopped descending again. It was an empowering and healing journey, but the same outcome: surrendering to the scalpel again. I had a huge gash where I allowed them to cut me open and take my baby from me. I kept my placenta for a placenta tree. They couldn't take that from me. But still… I wanted that vaginal birth experience. I wanted to say, "I trusted God and my body and it worked." I still feel compared to. Unworthy. I struggle with feeling like a real mom. Breastfeeding consumed me. I needed to be good at something after these experiences.

Healthy mom and baby is not a helpful comment. I didn't feel healthy after my homebirth cesarean or my CBAC. I didn't feel strong enough to be a good mom. I was devastated by what I perceived as a loss and a failure. I was grieving. I hurt so badly physically. I felt violated.

Have you seen pictures of how many layers they cut through to get to your baby? Have you ever had major surgery and then gone home without sleep or help or food or advice or support? Would you go back to work the same day as having your gallbladder removed? Would you schedule a knee replacement the same day as you were given a newborn baby? Stop and ask how I'm feeling before you make assumptions. Ask what I need and do it. Be supportive. Be objective. Hold your tongue. I'll be ready to talk when I'm ready and not before then.

Having a CBAC made me question the ability of my body. It made me wonder what would have happened to me if I lived in a time or place without access to cesareans. It has humbled me, broken me, strengthened me and changed me forever. My future births seem so complicated now. Handling young children at home after a CBAC is devastating. You can't pick them up and you're upset when they hit your incision because they don't know better. I've learned to treat myself as I would a cherished friend. Know that you did what you thought was best. You made the best decisions you could with the information you had. Know you are going to access a strength that you didn't know you were capable of.

None of Them Were Easy

I'm a newborn photographer and my clients love to share their birth stories, every good and bad thing. I struggle so much with this. They almost always ask how mine was because my son is about 8 months old. I hate to lie, so I'm truthful and let them know. I really don't like hearing about anyone's birth stories anymore. I hate hearing how easy it is. I have had three C-sections. None of them were easy. I tried so hard for a VBAC, and this last time around I was 41 weeks. I'll never feel like I was given the full chance to try. It had not even been 12 hours of active labor, and there were no signs of distress. My husband and I will never experience our baby being laid on my chest and those moments after that I always dreamed of.

Birth Is An Unknown

Initially, I felt broken and angry. Why me? Why again? What is wrong with my body? What makes others more worthy of a vaginal birth than me? This feels especially true when I hear that a person did an induction or something else typically viewed as "counterintuitive" for those hoping for a VBAC. I felt much more at peace with it after really coming to terms with it being a necessary procedure and that it wasn't my fault. Birth is an unknown, always.

I Feel Mixed Emotions

I felt horrible after my CBAC, like less than a real woman. I haven't been able to do something that women have been doing since the beginning of time. When I hear VBAC stories, I feel mixed emotions. I am both very happy and very envious. How were they able to do something I can't? Healthy mom and healthy baby isn't everything, and hearing that feels quite flippant and dismissive.

Both Experiences Were Very Good

I had an emergency C-section for my first because it was hospital policy for breech babies. I felt okay about being told I needed a C-section. The midwives and doctors worked really hard with me to get a VBAC the second time. I was sort of led to believe that my baby would flip. This was the only disappointing thing because he never budged. I felt like I had to try everything, when really I could have just settled into the pregnancy and my baby's choice. My desire for a vaginal birth was trumped by my babies' choice to be breech. I did not want to have a baby at home.

Near the end of my second pregnancy, when I was a bit down about him not flipping, I ran into a renowned midwife in our area who is the parent of my childhood best friend. She said to me, "Well, he just wants to hear your heart." Just those simple words and her nonchalance about my breech baby gave me so much reassurance that it is what it is. I loved that I labored with my first until the emergency C-section. I really wanted to experience at least that much. I was totally fine with my second C-section, as I tried everything to turn him. Both experiences were very good. I have very positive feelings about them both. I had a lot of support from family, husband, midwives, doctors and friends.

Everyone's Experience Is Different

My CBAC made me lose trust in healthcare providers. I did not educate myself on childbirth. I was afraid the worry would deprive me from enjoying my pregnancy and believed everyone's experience is different. It is, however, you learn from the mistakes you hear. Do not solely rely on healthcare providers. They let me push for four hours on my back, losing track of time because my baby and I seemed healthy. They should have been changing my position every 30 minutes to prevent the stall in labor. Please don't tell a cesarean mom that she should be happy that her baby is healthy and alive. No one is more grateful than she is for the good health of her baby. It's the trauma that she is struggling with, and the mourning of her dream, a planned vaginal birth, that was taken from her.

This Wasn't What I Wanted

I remember being wheeled down the hallway, into the elevator and then right outside the doors of the OR. The trip was so familiar, and I hated that I was back there. I was taken from the nice dark room and everything was so bright all of a sudden. The doctor greeted us by the OR doors, and I almost audibly groaned when I saw who it was: the doctor who I've only known to do C-sections on his patients. He was giddy and exuded confidence. He shook our hands and introduced himself, but I don't think he remembered that he helped with my C-section last time.

I was instantly uncomfortable again. He was so happy, and it made me angry. To be fair, I don't know how I would have preferred he acted. This was my baby's birthday after all, of course people were going to be happy.

I was happy I was about to meet my baby. I was also in shock and devastated. This wasn't what I wanted, and I wish that he would have shown some respect to that. I wanted so badly to prove that I could have a VBAC. I always perceived this doctor as somebody who didn't believe in women's bodies to give birth. Now he was helping me birth my baby and it felt like an "I told you so" situation. At that moment I thought to myself, "Why would you think you could ever deliver your baby naturally? You really are broken."

God Protected Us

I had a really normal first pregnancy with my son. At 39 weeks and 4 days, my water broke, but I wasn't in labor. We stayed home for a bit and called the doctor. He told me not to wait too long because I was at risk for infection. I thought I was in labor and having contractions, I just didn't know that I wasn't because I was a first time mom. Once we arrived, we were on a ticking time clock at the hospital. I just didn't dilate, no matter what they gave me. I got a foley bulb, then Pitocin, and then an epidural. Nothing got me contracting all that much. After 16 hours of Pitocin, my baby's heart rate dropped and didn't recover, so I had a C-section. I was in labor for 23 hours. I was convinced it was the hospital's fault, but now I'm not so sure. I feel more forgiving and understanding.

With my second I did all the things to get my natural birth. I switched providers twice and opted for an HBAC. I went to the Chiropractor every week from 8 weeks pregnant. I hired a doula. I did a crazy vitamin regimen, ate dates, despite me finding them disgusting, and drank red raspberry leaf tea. I did the Three Sisters of Balance with my husband every night. I did private hypnobirthing classes.

I was starting to feel like I was going into labor at 40 weeks. I would get a contraction every hour or two that was painful, and then it would go away. At 1:00 a.m., at 40 weeks and 3 days, I finally had real contractions on my own! I definitely thought that I would get my VBAC. I labored in bed until 5:00 a.m., and then woke my husband. They picked up after that, coming every 3-5 minutes. And then I thought my water broke. So we called the midwife and the doula and everyone came. But by 9:00 a.m. the contractions slowed. I took a short nap. My midwife said she would come back later and left the student midwife with us. My husband and I went to UPS to mail something and then to the grocery store. I had contractions in the grocery store. We also labored together a lot outside in our backyard and it was really lovely.

After that, the student midwife started me on a birth ball and a breast pump, plus gross tasting herbs to get things going again. My hubby and I didn't really want to continue doing it, so I told the midwife to come back later and we would reassess. Then my husband and I took a long hike (two hours) in the green belt behind our house. During the hike my contractions picked up again. I almost barfed on the way home from the pain. This was probably a mistake, given what was going to happen next, but we didn't know. I still thought I would have a natural birth. I really thought we would take a hike, have dinner, go to sleep and then I would get contractions again. I have a photo of me from that hike where I am 40 weeks pregnant, glowing, the sun is just right and I felt amazing. It's the last photo I have before everything really went awry.

After dinner, contractions were super intense and I really thought I was transitioning. I had to go to the bathroom. I lost the darkest mucus plug ever at this point. I was concerned about the color and called the midwife. It looked like black tar. She thought it was possibly meconium and came back to check on me. At this point, despite super intense contractions that were 3-5 minutes apart and lasting at least a minute over 2 hours, I still had not progressed past 3 cm. I had been at 3 cm and 80% effaced all day. My daughter's heart rate was racing. My midwife told us we had to transfer to the hospital because something wasn't right. My baby was super high in my pelvis and not engaging. My husband and I broke down in tears. We did not want to go at all. I have really intense sadness when I think about that moment. I also had not packed a proper hospital bag, and my doula had to help me. Lesson: always prepare a proper hospital bag! Man did it suck to pack while I was hysterical. But we packed up and got in the car and drove to the hospital.

I had the roughest car ride of my life. The contractions were insanely intense. In addition, I thought I was going to have a C-section the entire car ride, so it was a mix of sadness, intense crying, screaming in pain and staring out the window lifeless. We got to the hospital. They checked me there, no progress. They also confirmed that my water had not broken. Contractions were hellish by this point, and I was in labor 24 hours. They said they would give me an IV for fluids and that I could go home after that because I wasn't in "active labor" or I could stay if I wanted to. After the IV, the contractions were crazy intense, and I didn't want to get back in the car, so we stayed. I wanted pretty much anything but the car at that point. There was no progress and hellish contractions. I finally gave in for an epidural. I waited and waited because I was convinced the epidural would lead to another C-section. Once I gave in, the doctor took 1.5 hours to come. I actually thought I was going to die while waiting for him because I had given up at that point and couldn't manage the pain by breathing anymore. It was the most intense 90 minutes of my life. I have severe anxiety when I think back to that moment.

We got some sleep. I didn't progress though. My water broke and there was meconium. They put a peanut ball between my legs and told me they would wake me in a couple of hours to turn me onto my right side. When they turned me, I got this intense hot spot. It was worse than the contractions. They thought maybe my epidural wasn't working. So they gave me more and it sort of went away, but I could still feel it. At this point they started talking about Pitocin. But my daughter's heart rate wasn't doing so well, so they wanted to wait. We waited a bit and then my husband and I talked. At this point I was in labor for 32 hours. We decided it was time for a repeat C-section. The OB agreed and said she was willing to try one more thing, but that she didn't think it would work, and that after that we would be doing a C-section anyways.

It felt empowering to choose the C-section the second time. In addition, the hospital staff treated us well, explained everything and were respectful, despite us being a home birth transfer. I am really grateful for that.

We went to the OR. When they opened me, they immediately found meconium outside my uterus and all over my insides. My uterus had ruptured. They got my baby out and took over an hour to get me all sorted out after the fact. The hot spot was likely my uterine rupture, but the doctor said that the wound didn't look fresh and that I had probably been walking around with a tear for a while and didn't know it (probably those painful contractions leading up to actual labor).

My daughter's foot was wrapped three times by the cord and she couldn't descend. Apparently that saved her life, and my life, because had she descended, the rupture would have been way worse and possibly in my home. The weird part is, apparently my uterus had never healed properly from my first C-section. The muscles never went back together properly and the only thing holding my uterus together was the wall. The muscles had a space between them, and the wall had a bunch of scar tissue. The OB said it was super rare and she had never seen it before.

It was never in the cards for me to have a VBAC. Babies apparently get wrapped by the cord on their feet in the second trimester. My uterus was never going to hold together. I do feel like God protected me, and I also feel confused by all the chaos. I am not able to have more children, so I will never have a VBAC, and that makes me sad. I am also grateful for the family I do have. It pains me that both my births were bittersweet. But sometimes that is the card you get in life.

Worth It

Some days I feel like I failed because others around me tell me I took the "easy" way out. Little did they know most cesareans are only done when necessary. We didn't choose this route, it chose us. I had HELLP syndrome and my second child I only had preeclampsia close to HELLP, but without the platelet count and liver problems. I still wonder what it's like, what it would've been like to have a vaginal birth. It's okay. We're strong; we got this. All that pain was worth it. Look at that baby in front of you!

Birth Is the Entry Point

My water broke and I immediately went into hard and fast labor. We arrived at the hospital at 7 cm. I really thought my VBAC was going to happen. The nurse checked me, and each time my dilation increased. She finally told me that I was ready for the doctor, and I was ecstatic. The labor had been manageable, and I was ready to give birth.

The doctor came in to check me and said that the nurse was wrong and I was only 7 cm. The labor got intense after that. It was so intense that I begged for an epidural, but I never progressed after that. My baby started deceling. All that excitement, gone. There was just so much physical and emotional pain. I felt we did all we could in that moment. Looking back, I think we could have done more. But in the moment I felt that I made an informed decision and was able to ask for certain things to make it a gentle C-section, and that felt empowering.

I actually felt very empowered while having my CBAC. I felt I did everything possible to prepare for a VBAC. It seemed like it was going to happen, but labor got too intense and my baby started having a hard time. We made a community decision to opt for the C-section. Even though I felt empowered, the C-section surgery was very tough. I kept losing consciousness and felt like I couldn't inhale. I seemed to block that experience out immediately, but it was very traumatic for my husband. Although we were thinking about having a third child, after this trauma, we're likely not going to do this again. I feel so happy for the women who get their VBAC, but I can't understand why my body can't do it. I told myself that my body was made to do this, but I don't really believe that anymore. I have to address that my doctors labeled me as a failed TOLAC, and that was probably the most painful part, being labeled as a failure at birthing my baby.

Be proud of yourself for doing the best you could for your baby. Also remember that birth is the entry point, but there are a million more moments that will shape your baby's life. It's okay.

Find Peace in Your Story

I was angry. I was young, scared, and didn't know how to advocate for myself. I wish so much that I could go back and ask more questions. I strongly believe that I would not have been pushed into a C-section with my first if I hadn't been on Medicaid. It's hard to explain, but it's as if they did extra procedures and created made up issues just to bill it because they knew it would get paid. The level of care I received as an unmarried mother on Medicaid, compared to the care I received as a married, self-insured mother, was vastly different. Mind you these two experiences happened at the same hospital with the same partner less than 2 years apart.

I'm more angry about my first C-section because it led to my second, though I should be angry about that too. I was basically told that with everything that happened with my first it wasn't even safe to try for a VBAC, which was not true. Again, I can't help but feel like the provider took the "easy way out."

I'm about to have my fourth C-section, and I have to admit there are definitely some conveniences. I can choose when we have the baby, making childcare arrangements for the others MUCH easier. Recovery isn't "easy," but I've heard some serious horror stories about vaginal births that are by far worse than a CBAC. There is no tearing and everything down there pretty much stays intact. You're left with a nice scar on your tummy, but for the most part there aren't very many unknowns like there can be with VBACs. To a certain extent knowing what to expect is comforting.

There are pluses and minuses to both. You are still a mother that grew and birthed a baby, do not discount that. Find your peace within your story. It all happened exactly as it was supposed to happen. Comparison is the thief of happiness.

God Has a Plan

I have two children who were both born via cesarean section. With both pregnancies I was induced with Pitocin, and I was on it for 8 hours both times. Both times I had the same result: tons and tons of contractions with zero progress. I had no dilation, no dropping of the babies, nothing. I felt so defeated and like I had done something wrong.

God always has a plan. My first baby was face up, and the umbilical cord was around his neck so there could have been complications. With my second baby the umbilical cord was around his neck as well. So even though my babies didn't enter the world exactly as planned, I have two happy, healthy children. At first I felt defeated. I felt like I had failed in some way. Women everywhere have babies "the normal way" every day, so why couldn't I? I eventually stopped beating myself up about how my baby came into the world because I was holding a perfectly healthy baby. What more could I ask for? I feel disappointed in myself because I couldn't do it, but I'm always happy for anyone who doesn't have to undergo major surgery when having a baby. When I hear of someone who had a VBAC, my mind always goes through the what ifs and the what could have beens for myself.

For anyone going through this, I know it's not what you planned for, but holding a healthy baby in the end is the ultimate goal. Hold your head high, and don't beat yourself up too much because God has a plan, and even when it's hard, we have to trust Him.

The Pain Led Me to My Purpose

I had two stalled labors. I never got past 7 cm. For the longest time, I thought something must be structurally wrong with me because I had two births in a row where I didn't progress. I was told a vaginal birth would never happen for me because my pelvis was too small. I almost didn't try for my VBA2C because of that.

But I kept praying and searching, and the only thing that gave me peace was to try again. I'm on the other side of my mountain now, so it's easy for me to say, " Trust that there is purpose in this," but I remember how distraught and sad I was after my CBAC. I truly did feel broken, and it grieved me so much. I felt very alone, like no one understood me. It's okay if you feel sad about your birth. Whatever you are feeling right now is normal. Allow yourself to grieve. My biggest thing I want to communicate is that each birth is special and changes us. Even when things don't go as planned, God uses it to grow us. I honestly don't think that I would have had the courage to walk the path that I'm on now if not for my first C-section and CBAC. Truly, I don't. The pain led me to my purpose.

Breech Babies

Of course there had to be a chapter dedicated to breech baby stories, as I have had two breech babies myself. This book is called "Variations of Normal," and breech presentation is exactly that! Having a breech baby is a unique experience. Some mothers feel that they have no option other than having a cesarean that they don't want, while others leave the hospital system to birth their babies at home. No matter what a mother chooses when it comes to delivering a breech baby, she should feel supported and have access to a safe birth.

Change of Plans

I found out during an ultrasound at 41 weeks 5 days that my second baby was breech. Having a breech baby made me ineligible for my planned home water birth. The midwives in my area are not allowed to deliver known breech babies. I was terrified. The one and only thing about birth that scared me was a C-section.

I attempted to find a vaginal breech provider, but the only one in my area was on leave. No one else presented it as an option. My biggest regret was not fighting harder to find one. My C-section was scheduled for Monday, but I went into labor at 3:00 a.m. on Sunday. We headed to the hospital when I determined I was in labor, around 7:30 a.m.

My second son was born at 10:25 a.m. I was in tears because everyone else could see him except for me. It was a devastating change of plans that I still struggle with some days. I felt ashamed and defeated that I didn't fight harder. I struggled with my recovery emotionally because I was so sad about the outcome of my birth. I want all providers to be comfortable with vaginal breech birth. I feel strongly that all mothers should be presented with all options to decide for themselves.

No Other Choice

There is a very helpless feeling when you are told that your baby is breech and a C-section is needed. My baby was also diagnosed with IUGR, and I had low fluid, so I was not a candidate to manually flip. At 36 weeks and 4 days my water broke at home while doing laundry. My first reaction was to cry because I knew it meant I had to have a C-section. The sonogram two days prior showed my baby girl was breech. I cried the whole drive to the hospital and was asked 100 times what was wrong and if I was okay. I just did not want a C-section, but I had no other choice. Instead of the excitement of my first baby coming, I was overwhelmed with sadness of having to birth her from a C-section. Obviously I was excited to meet her and prayed that she was healthy, but the emotions of having to have a C-section took over. I wanted to experience labor and birth. I felt like that was all taken from me.

Insanely Stressful

My midwives were supportive and said that I was a good candidate for a vaginal breech birth since I already had one baby born vaginally. They just couldn't do it because they had no experience. I had to find another midwife who was on board. All of the OBs I talked to made me feel scared and like I was making the wrong choice. The whole situation leading up to his birth was insanely stressful. It should not be like that. Women should not have to fight for something their bodies can do. We just need skilled providers who can help if it is needed. I am so happy I chose a vaginal delivery; I was able to go home right away and I had an easy recovery.

It Was Traumatic

I was in the middle of pushing when it was discovered that my baby was in the breech position. I'm a labor/ delivery nurse, and we had recently seen a breech birthing center transfer who died. When they told me my baby was breech, I immediately thought my baby was going to die while they transferred me across the street to the hospital from my birthing center. It was a horribly traumatic 15 minutes because of my own prior experiences. Physically, my breech delivery was easier than my first, head-presenting delivery. But emotionally, it was very traumatic because of my prior knowledge and experience. I have since done a lot of healing with therapy and more research, and I think I was likely the best possible candidate for a breech delivery. Some of the trauma might have been avoided if we didn't have such a negative mindset about breech deliveries.

Lots of Hoops to Jump Through

With my first I was told by my family doctor, and later my OB, that I would most likely need a cesarean. I was devastated. I felt like I had lost all power over my birth process. I felt robbed of my birth experience. I wound up having vaginal births with both babies. The actual births made me feel strong, in control, and powerful. It was disappointing that I had to fight to get it with my first, causing so much stress leading up to the event. There were lots of hoops to jump through. The ninth month was not what it should have been.

With my second birth, I just said "F- it" to the OB's opinion and everyone who didn't support my vaginal breech birth. I knew I could do it and it would be great. While I do not think all medical intervention is bad, the only issues that arose in either of my births was from a medical intervention. I had a planned mandatory episiotomy with my first birth that was stitched badly and led to many other issues. It was ridiculous that they said this was "required." My body clearly wants to, and can, deliver breech babies. I shouldn't have been made to feel like it was a medical issue.

I Cried Tears of Joy

The birth was terrible and didn't go as planned. My baby was breech, but I saw a chiropractor that specializes in pregnancies and the Webster's Technique. I did inversions, stayed super active, bought books on how to flip a breech baby, but nothing worked.

At 36 weeks I went in for my last ultrasound and routine check up. They sent me over to the hospital for labs because I had preeclampsia and my blood pressure was super high. I didn't end up leaving, and my baby was still breech. I was admitted to the hospital at 12:30, and at 3:52 my son was born via C-section. Nothing about his birth was beautiful and magical like I expected it to be.

As soon as they pulled him out it was silent. The nurses and doctors were talking about NICU, and I could hear the panic in their voices. He had yet to let out a cry, so I started bawling, thinking something was wrong. He had the umbilical cord wrapped around his neck twice. Finally, I heard his cry, and for the first time throughout the whole process, I cried tears of joy. I hated that I didn't have the immediate skin to skin contact and that he got rolled back into the room while I laid on the table getting stitched back up. But once I got to hold him and see his little face, I knew I would love him forever and be the best mommy I could be.

Empowered

I had an unassisted homebirth 12 years ago with our first born. Then we had three miscarriages, which were very heartbreaking, so I decided that I didn't want another child because it's just too traumatic to go through these sad situations. A few months after the last miscarriage I started showing signs of pregnancy. I didn't know how to handle it. I was shocked and didn't want to get too excited too quickly and just took every day as it came. We went for our 8 week check up and were told that we were actually 9 weeks pregnant already and that the fetus looked very strong and like it was a good pregnancy. We still waited a few weeks before we told people. The 12 week mark came, and we started telling people, but we were still a bit scared to get too excited. At 18 weeks I stopped going to the gynecologist, as I wanted a home birth again like the first time.

At 30 weeks we went to find a midwife that could assist us this time, as we weren't too sure what we actually wanted. By 36 weeks we found out that our baby boy was breech. We went to see a gynecologist, and she suggested a C-section by 39 weeks. I left there knowing that it was not what we wanted. We wanted a natural birth and that was it. In the following weeks we tried everything to help our baby spin. At 38 weeks I went for another check up and second opinion by another gynecologist, and he suggested I go book my bed straight away for a C-section on the 19th of March, as our baby was still a complete breech. My heart was shattered.

I started to feel very depressed about the C-section, so the following day when I woke up I said to my husband, "I just can't go through with the C-section." He confirmed the same feeling and said whatever I decide to do he would support me. That same morning my aunt, who is a doula, phoned me and we had a good chat. She confirmed that I could do it, as God created our bodies to be able to give birth, breech or not breech.

I phoned the doctor's office and cancelled the C-section. I also told my midwife that I needed some time to think of what I needed to do, as I felt she didn't keep my interests at heart with what I wanted, and our paths separated. She would check every now and then to see if I decided to go through with the C-section that was suggested, and I just kept telling her that it's not what I want. The gynocologist was also not very happy. We started to research breech births and we saw that it is possible. We had a few confirmations from other people over the next few weeks, and the research didn't stop.

The estimated due date was the 30th of March. The day came and went. So did the next few days after that, and a C-section started to sound not too bad by the 3rd of April. The 4th of April I woke up at 2:08 in the morning with feelings of contractions. I downloaded an app on my phone to time the contractions. By 5:00 a.m. I asked my hubby to run me a bath. I could feel the contractions were here to stay. Hubby and my mom started prepping everything for the birth in our room. I got to a point where the fear took over a bit again, and I thought maybe we should go to the hospital. With the lockdown, I didn't want to expose my newborn to all those germs, so I decided to push through and keep my focus on what my heart wanted.

By 10:00 a.m. I told my husband that I would like to have another bath, as it helped for pain relief. While I was in the bath, my water broke, so then the contractions really started to be extra strong. By 1:45 p.m. my body started to push, so I got on all fours on the floor where we prepared the spot for birth. After a few strong contractions, one foot fell out and soon after the bum, and the other foot followed. With the next contraction I focused on pushing as hard as I could to get the body through, so the right arm fell out, and the left shoulder got stuck.

Luckily my mom knew exactly what to do, so she dislodged the left arm and shoulder. The next contraction I knew I had to get the head out no matter what. So I put my all into that push and the head came through. My breech baby dropped to the mattress in a completely hands off birth. He was born at 2:10 p.m. He wasn't breathing for a few seconds or so, but he was still connected to the life line, so I wasn't too worried. I just rubbed and encouraged him to breathe and look at us. His eyes opened and he took his first breath. We were all so overwhelmed with joy.

We knew God was part of this birth and pregnancy from day one, and He will never let go of you as long as you keep your faith. We never once lost our faith and put the whole pregnancy and birth in His hands. Our baby boy ended up in our lives, and we are so in love and empowered that we went against all medical advice and followed our hearts and leaned on God to guide us. We thank God every day for His guiding hand in all we do and that He never disappoints.

Birth Was Quick

I am really glad I never knew she was breech during pregnancy. I am so pleased I never had the scaremongering and pressure put on me about what was best for my baby. I went into labor when my body was ready. My body did its thing and birthed her beautifully. I am very happy to have found out that she was breech when her little bottom appeared rather than her head. The midwife arrived just in time. It was an amazing, breech vaginal birth at home, undiagnosed. This was my first baby, so I had nothing to compare it to in terms of what I was feeling. Labor was quick; birth was quick. It was definitely easier and quicker than the birth of my second baby, who was head down. I would very happily give birth vaginally to a breech baby again.

My Wishes Weren't Respected

I was devastated when I found out my baby was breech. I had been planning on delivering naturally at a birth center, but I was risked out of their care with a breech baby. I was very upset when I was told I would need a C-section. I cried every day from finding out at 36 weeks, to 39 weeks when my water broke on its own. I tried everything to flip my baby around: ECV (which was extremely painful), Spinning Babies, acupuncture and moxibustion, seeing a chiropractor every day, homeopathic pulsatilla, and even lying on an ironing board with frozen peas on the top of my belly and a heating pad on the bottom.

By the time my water broke, I was already resigned to my cesarean fate. That didn't make my birthing experience easier to handle. My wishes weren't respected multiple times, and I felt bullied. Not all staff members were like this, but enough of them were to make an impression. It was traumatic, and I still regret making that choice today. The amount of manipulation and fear used by medical professionals is disgusting. I asked my midwife at one point if there was any way I could have this baby vaginally. She said to me, "If you show up to the hospital 10 centimeters and pushing. But if you do that, your baby could die." I know now that she was wrong. There are competent professionals in my area who support and have experience with delivering breech. There are always alternative options, and if you don't like what you hear, get a second, third, or fourth opinion. Breech is a variation of normal, and if my subsequent children are breech, I will not be consenting to another cesarean.

They Were Clueless

I woke up in the morning the day before I delivered, called my work to tell them I was in labor, and rested all morning. In the early afternoon, I went to my regular OB appointment. I was told that I was, indeed, in labor and to go back home to labor until my contractions were more frequent and closer together. About 9:00 p.m., I told my husband that I was ready to go in. He is from Southeast Asia, and he and his siblings were all born at home into the hands of their father. He told me that I would feel better if I took a hot shower. He was right! When I got dressed, I was ready to leave, but he told me I looked tired and I would probably feel better after a nap. Again, he was right! I slept between contractions for about four hours.

When I woke my contractions were to the point I could not catch my breath and there was not much of a break from one to the next. When I arrived at the hospital, the nurse checked my cervix, and praised me for being already dilated to 4 cm. I was LIVID! I really thought I was ready to deliver, but I had a long way to go. So I did everything I could to encourage my contractions to come. I sat up, walked to the bathroom, got on my hands and knees, and tried constant movement.

After about four hours, the nurse came in to check dilation again, and the water broke. There was meconium in the water and the nurse's eyes got really wide. DON'T PUSH, she warned. I immediately had the urge to push. Puffing out my cheeks, I did everything possible to slow down the baby's birth while we waited for the doctor to arrive. The nurse told us that the baby would likely be born via C-section, but when the doctor arrived 20 minutes later, he soon realized it was too late for surgery. They wheeled me into the delivery room and immediately the room filled with other doctors and nurses who were interested in witnessing the birth. My husband helped me sit up while I pushed the baby out in 3 contractions. He had a huge bruise on his butt, but was otherwise pink and perfect. He delivered frank breech, face forward, with his feet next to his ears at 7 lb, 1 oz.

The nurse who attended my breech birth was also present at my other two (cephalic) deliveries. She was instrumental in keeping the other nurses from being bothersome while I labored with my other two. "She knows what she's doing, you can leave her alone." I'm so grateful. I am thankful that my care providers were clueless about the position prior to my water breaking and second stage of labor. Not only did that give me the opportunity to push my baby out vaginally, it also gave an opportunity for many hospital personnel to witness a non-medicated vaginal breech birth.

I Felt Disconnected

I felt helpless. A cesarean was the last thing I wanted. I was worried about major abdominal surgery. I put off scheduling anything until the last moment because I was reluctant for it to be true. I was worried I would resent my baby. I ended up being upset with the doctor for not providing any other options. I felt disconnected from my cesarean breech delivery. My water broke spontaneously a couple weeks early. From rupture to delivery, it was less than two hours. I didn't have time to process anything, as I was still in denial about the way she would be entering the world. Breech is a variation of normal, and women should not feel optionless and unsupported when it comes to how they can birth their baby.

It Was a Great Experience

My second baby was breech for most of the pregnancy. I always felt kicks down very low near my panty line and out the sides of my belly. My doctor suggested a C-section if he stayed breech, but I asked to be referred to an OB who supported vaginal breech birth. I spent weeks worrying about deciding on a C-section or having a natural birth, and not many people in my family were supportive of a natural birth. We were very lucky in our town to have three OBs who would deliver breech. The doctor I met with was absolutely amazing. He was full of information and very supportive. He really helped make me feel at ease with a natural birth.

I went into labor around 36 weeks and headed to the hospital. All of the nurses and doctors at our hospital were very supportive. They presented all of our options with no judgment or suggestions. Labor progressed fairly quickly, but they did have to break my water. Around 11 hours into labor, I still wasn't feeling pressure as my baby hadn't fully engaged, so the doctor recommended we head to the OR (where they deliver all breech babies in case things take a turn). Once in the OR, we started to push. My baby was born in less than 10 minutes of pushing! It felt easier than my first labor, which was a head down baby. We were both healthy and had a great experience. If I had another breech baby, I would do the exact same thing.

I Knew In My Heart I Could Do It

I made an appointment for a C-section three times, but I canceled them all and had her at home. I had two ECVs. The second one fractured my baby's skull, but we didn't know until after birth. I did Webster's certified chiropractor, Spinning Babies, laying inverted, hot and cold on my belly, flashlight, music, took pulsatilla, acupuncture with moxibustion, handstands in water... You name it, I did it! I found my midwife at 39 weeks after the hospital said I couldn't have a vaginal breech birth there. Thank God I found someone to help me! I didn't deliver until 42+2. My baby was 9 lbs 12 oz! I was scared, but just knew in my heart I could deliver vaginally after having 3 cephalic vaginal births. It would have been perfect if not for the skull fracture, the surgery to correct it, and a four day NICU stay.

Breech with Multiples

It was devastating to me. Once it was confirmed that both babies had turned breech, my entire team no longer felt comfortable, or that it was safe, for me to still have a homebirth. There was only one practicing physician at one hospital that was comfortable doing a breech extraction, under the circumstances that baby A was head down and baby B was Frank breech. I had no other options after my ultrasound at 39 weeks, unless I were to attempt an unassisted birth, which was not a comfortable option for me.

It is so vitally important to find providers that are experienced, confident and comfortable with breech birth, particularly if you're pregnant with multiples. I wish I had a more reliable and experienced team of midwives when we found out both babies were breech. I also wish I had joined the Coalition for Breech Birth sooner. I would have had more information to advocate for myself, and I possibly could have found another provider upon short notice who would have honored my home birth.

The place we had my ultrasound done was at perinatal (intended for "high risk" pregnancies, which multiples fell under). They are NOT used to seeing twin moms get to nearly 40 weeks, and they found reasons to be concerned in my ultrasound that ended up being false post birth. The false pieces of information were that baby A had meconium in their fluid, that my placentas were starting to calcify, and that baby A was a footling breech (baby A was not a true footling breech, and that small piece of information changed so much for me and my options). Lastly, their guesstimate of babies' weights were at least a pound off.

I Was Scared

I was very far along in labor (almost ready to push). They had not checked me, and my water did not break until the last minute. I was exhausted, and my only knowledge of breech was that you had to have a

C-section. So I was delirious, as I was in transition with no medication/no epidural, and I kept asking if I was going to have to have a C-section. I was not getting an answer, as the midwife was trying to call the OB to come.

I was so confused and scared, and I seriously thought I was going to die. I kept asking if either I or the baby was going to die. I wound up delivering vaginally. On my second breech baby, I was totally prepared and just nervous about having another 4th degree tear. The first birth was super scary. I didn't even care when my baby was born. It was so sad. The second was incredible, and I loved watching as her grey little body came out and up onto my belly.

It Was Unexpected

I found out my first baby was breech when I was pushing, so there was no way to go but to push him out. If I had found out sooner with my first, I would have had to do a C-section, which would have absolutely destroyed me. My second baby was also breech, but didn't find out until I was in labor. She flipped because she had been head down the week before. I was shocked, but there was nothing I could do about it. She was a double footling breech. I was in a different state for my second, and the midwives said that since I'd given birth to a breech baby before that they would be okay with it if the second baby was breech. My first vaginal breech I felt like a superhero, like I could conquer the world. I felt amazing. The second vaginal breech delivery was very fast, unexpected, and somewhat traumatizing since I gave birth in the L&D waiting room.

A Toll on My Mental Health

At first, I was determined to get my baby to flip. I was stressed due to the fact I could no longer deliver her at the out of hospital birth center and would need to find a new provider. Overall, the whole last 4 weeks (turned out closer to 6 weeks because she arrived past her due date) were incredibly stressful and took a toll on my mental and physical health. Up until then, the pregnancy was lovely.

My midwives provided me with all the information they knew on how to flip babies. Thankfully, via their referrals and my amazing doula, I was able to find two providers whose first choice was not a cesarean. One provider told me cesarean only, though. I did not want a cesarean, and I knew I could continue to find other options. So it didn't really bother me as much as it could have. I had a vaginal birth at a hospital with a provider who was

72

doing vaginal breech births back in the 80s/ 90s, when it was commonplace. He was great and did not question my choice at all.

The only thing I did not love about the experience was having to push in the operating room while lying on my back. I would have preferred kneeling on all fours. But by the time we found this doctor and worked it all out, in the moment of laboring and delivery, I was simply done fighting for things. I was happy to get to deliver vaginally with essentially no intervention. Although I did end up having to be induced, which was not ideal, but it went fine and didn't impact my delivery experience on the whole. I will mention that I hated the post delivery period in a hospital. Had I been able to deliver at the birth center out of hospital, I would have been home in 8 hours or less. There would have been much less interruption and stress.

I dealt with some pretty awful pediatric providers who were arrogant, not following evidence based practices, and going against hospital protocol in their recommendations. I had to fight them a lot to get out of there ASAP and, in the end, my lovely daughter had zero issues that they thought I was being a neglectful parent about. Literally zero issues. Honestly, I should consider reporting them, especially one of them. It made the whole hospital experience more traumatic and worse than it needed to be. The nurses were lovely, though. And a couple did help me deal with the pediatric providers.

Honestly, if I could do it all over again, I would not stress so much about doing all the things I did to try to flip her. I think, in the end, it made it more stressful and worse. Had I been less tense and stressed maybe the outcome would have been different. However, I'm grateful there are local providers who still do vaginal breech deliveries. Also, the delivery itself did not feel any different than my head down delivery. Pushing a baby out is pushing a baby out!

No Other Options

I was nervous. My first breech baby was my third child. My other two were head down by 20 weeks. So when 20 weeks came and went and my third was still breech, I figured she wasn't moving. I was absolutely terrified. I had two vaginal births prior. My first with an epidural, and my second all natural. I had planned my birth from start to finish, and a C-section was absolutely not in that plan.

I tried Spinning Babies, bouncing on a ball, and chiropractic care. I asked for an ECV, but my doctor stated that he doesn't do those. So I had a C-section, and it felt forced. It felt like I had no other option or my baby would die. It traumatized me and broke my heart that my last birth was one that I felt like I had no voice or say in. I just wish I wouldn't have been afraid to advocate for myself. Breech is a variation of normal.

It Wasn't a Good Experience

I tried pretty much everything to turn my baby around. Ironically I had been doing prenatal yoga, spinning babies and seeing a Webster Certified Chiropractor my whole pregnancy, not because I was concerned about breech, but I just wanted a better birth experience. I had two failed ECVs, even one with an epidural. They got him to turn, but as soon as they let go, he flipped right back to Frank breech. My midwife provided vaginal breech birth as an option if I wanted, but it was the doctors at the hospital who all tried to scare me out of trying vaginal. One doctor even said, "If anything goes wrong, you will wake up in the basement," referring to the recovery area for emergency cesarean. I was glad I didn't need a cesarean, but it certainly wasn't a good experience. I did not feel respected or supported by the doctors. I had to deliver in the OR "just in case," and they forced me onto my back after I said no. They did all the maneuvers without giving him a chance to be born hands off. They immediately cut the cord because he was slow to develop reflexes, but all they did was move him to the warmer and repeatedly dropped his arms until his startle reflex kicked in.

Trust Your Instincts

I had a 14 hour vaginal breech birth. At the time I felt very empowered and supported. I had a 4th degree tear and a rough recovery, but no regrets. In retrospect I wish I had pushed back a bit on the birthing position, but I knew that OB was my only option, and he really was quite amazing. I feel fortunate to have had access to a supportive birth care provider. I work in the birth industry and have seen success with chiropractic, acupuncture, Spinning Babies, all of it. But at the end of the day, for some babies, breech is their optimal fetal position. Trust yours and your baby's instincts. My daughter is not stubborn, but she does have her own way of doing things. It started at birth! She listens to her heart and gut, and they don't lead her astray. I listened to my heart and gut, and I have a beautiful birth story.

Defeated

I initially felt defeated, as a cesarean wasn't the birth I planned for. I'm more at peace with it now, but I'm afraid to have another breech baby in the future. My baby had issues with low amniotic fluid from 28 weeks. His position would go from transverse to breech. I was always told that my baby had time to turn, so I didn't do any interventions until 35 weeks. I had an ECV done at 38 weeks, and it failed. It nearly ended in a C-section because my baby's heart rate drastically dropped. I felt defeated because I felt that the ECV was my last shot. I went in for my scheduled C-section a week later at 39 weeks.

I mourned a vaginal birth for a while and even felt empowered to have a VBAC in the future, but I'm just not sure how I feel about a VBAC. It sounds like a lot of work to try to have one. I'm hoping I change my mind in the future, but for now I'm just afraid of being pregnant again because of the things I went through during my last pregnancy. Personally, I wish I found a provider that allowed breech vaginal deliveries. I loved my provider, but I wish they had options for a breech vaginal delivery.

It Gave Me Confidence

My experience with having had two vaginal breech births has made me a better woman. I give most of the credit for this to my midwife, who was with me during both my pregnancies and births. Her education and guidance, combined with her knowledge and experience, gave me the confidence to attempt a vaginal breech birth both times. I made the right decision for myself and my children, and I can honestly say that I absolutely loved giving birth! I am saddened when I think that I would not have birthed this way if I would have been under the care of a different hospital. That is what needs to change! Women deserve to have access to health care professionals that are well versed in facilitating variations of normal, such as breech presentation, safely.

I Tried Everything

I had planned an all natural community birth at a stand alone birth center. However, due to my state's laws, my midwives could not perform a breech delivery, which also meant I could not birth at my birth center. I found out at 35 weeks that if my baby did not turn, I would be forced into a hospital and cesarean birth. We tried an ECV five times, and they all failed. I tried everything to turn my baby.

I wound up with a cesarean. I felt hopeless and frustrated by this. In my city there were only two doctors trained in breech vaginal births. One retired a few months prior to my delivery, and the second wouldn't take a late transfer of care. This meant I had to have a C-section. At my C-section, the doctor I had scheduled my surgery with wasn't on call the night I went into labor. This meant I had a complete stranger who didn't listen to my needs, wants, or choices. She even took phone calls during my surgery!

I Still Feel a Disconnect

My midwife suggested various options, and her partner is a breech trained midwife. Later we found out the hospital didn't "support" a vaginal breech birth, and I was made to feel unsafe, so I opted for an "elective" C-section. I had a cesarean and felt, and still feel, like I have missed out on what it feels like to give birth. I don't feel like I actually birthed my baby girl. When I look at her sometimes I still feel a disconnect. I am not sure if having a vaginal birth would have made a difference, of course. It's a strange feeling and very hard to describe. I developed postpartum depression, and even though there were numerous factors at play, not having the birth experience that I had hoped for played a major part. It took me quite a while to bond with her. I never experienced the "high of love hormones" or a sense of achievement or pride with her birth.

It has been a difficult road for me personally. It kind of felt like the way she was positioned isn't normal. I still feel sad about it all, especially when other moms talk about going into labor and having this powerful experience when I had none of that. I really wish providers would become skilled again to deliver breech so that women can feel safe, supported, and empowered, no matter their decision on how to give birth. It should be the mother's choice how she wants to give birth, and at the moment hospitals have policies in place where that choice is taken away by fear and untrained and unsupportive providers.

Birth Trauma

There are many forms of trauma. Trauma can be the result of a life threatening event, birth-related injury, past assault, how the mother was treated during the birth, or anything else the mother deems as traumatic. Pregnancy and birth have a profound impact on mothers, especially with a trauma history. It affects them on a physical, mental and emotional level. The act of childbirth in itself can be a trigger that brings flashbacks of a past assault or dissociation. Some mothers had procedures done to them during birth without their consent, while others walked away from their experience with an injury. Trauma also has an impact on partners, doulas and medical providers. It is important to hold space for these individuals as they tell their stories.

The Birth Plan

There were a lot of things that were triggering to my past sexual assault during my pregnancy and birth: the provider's hands measuring my belly, the vaginal exams, the physical sensations of my baby moving. All of it was deeply upsetting. With my first pregnancy I wrote an excessive birth plan. I desperately wanted to be in control and not to feel like a victim again. Pregnancy and birth opened old wounds that I wished I could forget.

Making a Small Difference

I'm an OB nurse. I went to nursing school after having to fight like hell for my right to have a VBAC. I wanted to be there for other women like me. I wanted to help change things in the birthing world. I feel like I'm making a small difference on a patient to patient basis, but It's definitely not the big change that I hoped for. I feel that it's impossible for nurses at my hospital to create positive change. Nothing ever comes from nurses filing complaints against doctors. The most abusive obstetrician at my hospital is the chief of OB. He is at the top of the "chain of command," and there is no recourse for nurses who report the wrong being done. If more patients report the abuse that's being done, maybe things will change.

Every Stitch

The medical personnel didn't tell me what they were doing as they were doing it. At one point it felt like they were pushing my baby back inside of me. The doctor shoved his entire hand inside of me, and to this day I still don't know why. Afterwards, they stitched my episiotomy repair without any medication. Because I was on Medicaid, they had student doctors taking turns and learning how to stitch me up. I felt every stitch. I could hear the head doctor saying, "You're doing that wrong; you're going through the muscle!" The entire time my husband was recording it on the tape recorder. I was shaking uncontrollably, and my baby was on the other side of the room crying. I told my husband to go to her. When I told the doctor what I was feeling, he said, "You're not feeling a thing."

Disempowered

During my cesarean I felt disempowered, heartbroken, bullied, trapped and scared. I was in a domestic violence marriage and had a toddler. I was fearful for my ability to function post surgery and to keep myself and my kids safe. It was a horrific experience. I've been diagnosed with PTSD and anxiety as a result.

My Only Delivery Was Traumatizing

I previously had an issue with abnormal cells in my cervix when I was 18, and I saw a specialist in Omaha that I absolutely loved. But when I got pregnant at 18, I couldn't afford to go to Omaha for frequent visits for my pregnancy and had to settle with doctors in town. My doctor in Omaha told me there was no way I would be able to have a natural birth because my hips were too small and he believed that it would be difficult. The doctors in town told me that natural delivery wouldn't be an issue. I should have listened to my specialist and found a way to have him as my labor and delivery doctor.

I walked around for the entire month of August 2008 at 4 cm dilated, and I saw two different doctors because one of mine was on vacation. One of them said I wouldn't make it to my due date at the end of August. On August the 22nd I was about 6 cm dilated, and they thought I was going to give birth that day, so they admitted me to the hospital. I was there all day. They released me in the evening because I hadn't progressed, but I was having contractions. I made an appointment for Monday morning to be induced. My grandmother flew in from Vegas at the last minute and arrived on Saturday. She believed in all those old wives tales and had me drink Castor oil. That was disgusting! I proceeded to have frequent bowel movements the rest of the day and the next. That was fun. Not.

Monday I woke up about 12:30 in the morning with severe back pain, and I decided to stand in the hot shower for about an hour. I laid on the couch and timed my contractions. They were getting really close together, so I went to the hospital (drove myself) and I was in active labor. I managed to get a little bit of rest before full blown labor. The doctor came in and broke my water, even though they knew that he was sunny side up. They tried all these fancy moves to try and get him to turn after they broke my water, which made no sense because now he didn't have a way to turn easily. The pain was so severe from the contractions that it felt like my lower back was going to break. It hurt so bad. It wasn't even pain in the front; it was pain in the back, which I learned was back labor. Oh, the joys of back labor. They warned in my labor classes that back labor was the worst type of labor, and, of course, that was the labor that I had. I sat on a little bouncing ball and bounced, I walked the halls, and I had the best labor and delivery nurse who would rub my back for me.

Eventually they let me have an epidural, and I managed to fall asleep for a couple hours because everything was numb. Then, for some reason, the epidural wore off, and no matter how many times I hit that damn button, it didn't work at all for the rest of my labor. I finally told them that I felt like I had to poop, and they refused to check me and said that I wasn't ready to push. I was adamant that I was going to poop myself, and they finally checked me and said that I was ready to push. They had me pushing on my knees. Then they had me pushing with a pull-up bar. And finally they had me pushing the traditional way. He wasn't budging at all. He was stuck in my birth canal. I remember my grandmother saying that she could see a baseball-sized portion of his head and that she had seen enough of me to last a lifetime. That was the only time in my life that I ever threw profanities at my grandmother, and I will never do it again.

The pain was so immense after 2 ½ hours of pushing and him not going anywhere. They checked on him, and they said that he was fine, but I was not okay. I remember them telling me that I needed to have an emergency C-section, and they asked me to sign a paper. I was so out of it from the amount of pain and exhaustion that I asked if my mom could sign it. They told me that since I was an adult, I would have to sign it. I remember just dragging the pen across the page, not even trying to make a signature, because I hurt so much and wanted to get this over with. All of my friends and family that were waiting for me to have the baby had left because my screams were scaring them. It was that painful. I remember going into the OR and they were poking my belly and asking if I could feel it. I said to them, "No shit!" My epidural wasn't working, what did they expect? And they kept trying to pump more meds through my epidural line, which clearly wasn't working. I was so uncomfortable from the contractions that I couldn't focus. They finally said that they would have to completely sedate me in order to get my son out.

I remember waking up sometime in the evening, and it was dark. Mind you, my son was born at 3:40 in the afternoon, in the middle of summer, when it was daylight until 9:30 in the evening. I really had to go to the bathroom when I woke up, and they said I had a catheter and just let it go. That was weird. Then they asked if I wanted to meet my son, and they put him in my arms, and I remember being so out of it still that I looked at him like, "What the heck is this?" I had absolutely no emotion, which was devastating because I had just given birth. You would expect a mother to be happy. I only saw my son for a little bit, and someone took a couple pictures, then they took him away and I went back to sleep. The next day I woke up, and they moved me to a different room because I was freezing the night before. Apparently the heat didn't work in that room, and the air conditioning worked too well. I asked them about breastfeeding, and they told me that it was too late because they had already started him on a bottle, so he wouldn't take it now. They didn't even try. I was kind of sad because I didn't plan on formula feeding.

The next few days went by as a blur. I ended up being a freaking robot, taking care of my son for weeks by myself. Then postpartum hit like a ton of bricks. I didn't know what to do. I didn't have a ton of support, and I remember it was really early in the morning when I finally hit my breaking point. I called my mom and told her that she would have to take him because I couldn't do it. I had been spiraling back into alcoholism and severe depression. I was committed to the hospital, where I only had to stay a couple days because I played a good story, and they didn't believe anything was wrong with me, so they let me out. I struggled with alcoholism for several months, all the while continuing to go to my mom's house, trying to help take care of this child that felt like he was my brother and not my son.

I firmly believe that my labor led to my severe postpartum depression and didn't allow for me to create that bond with my son when he was first born. I enjoyed pregnancy, even though the first part was difficult, but I really did enjoy it. A few years ago I ended up having to have a hysterectomy due to health problems. I never did get to have another child where I could actually enjoy labor and delivery, with someone to help me through everything, which is really devastating considering the only labor and delivery I had was traumatizing. It still bothers me 12 years later.

Witnessing Trauma

As a doula I've seen my clients go through fear and manipulation, belittling, unconsented episiotomies, three day long inductions, pulling at placentas, and unconsented cord clamping. I feel that the hospital system harms women everyday, and I personally felt convicted that I was being complicit in that abuse by being there. I only attend planned home births now because of the trauma I witnessed.

I Was Put Completely Under

I had preeclampsia and my blood pressure was 144/120. I had to have an emergency C-section. I was more scared of the epidural than anything. First, they tried the epidural after multiple sticks without success. Then they tried the spinal tap, but they had the same issue. They kept hitting the nerve in my spine because when I crashed my car at 19, I crushed my lower vertebrae. The doctor said the only way I'd have my baby was to be put completely under anesthesia.

When I woke up, they were scared that I would have seizures. I had a spinal headache as a side effect of the epidural and spinal tap together. They had to do a blood patch, which didn't have any effect. My first week as a mom meant me laying down 90% of the time because if I sat up, the pain felt like my head would explode. This was not the feeling I wanted, but I did get a lot of cuddles and skin to skin time with my baby.

These Cases Stick with You

Most of us genuinely care for our patients and we're not trying to be the "bad guys." I've seen seemingly normal deliveries go south in an instant.

I'm trying to be more conscious of how these experiences have affected me, and how they affect my decisions during other births. It's hard not to make decisions out of fear when I think of the tragedies I've seen. These cases stick with you.

I Felt Robbed

With my third child, I thought I was an old pro. I had successfully delivered two children previously with no pain meds, and they were very easy deliveries, just an hour or two long. When I went into labor with my third child, I was sick and went to the hospital while having contractions. After a while they weren't getting anywhere, so they decided to break my water. They would only give me so much time after my water broke, and then they were going to want to do a C-section.

I was not progressing, so they took an x-ray and saw that my baby's position was in a way that he was not going to come out. They told me that they were getting the room ready for me to have a C-section at 8 o'clock. The doctor wanted to get it done that night because he was going to play golf the next day. I was silently terrified, trying to be brave. I was also disappointed because my 16 year old daughter was originally going to be there at the birth.

They tried to give me a catheter before my spinal, and the nurse wasn't getting it because she had never done one before. The other nurse was just talking her through it instead of taking over for her. Then they wheeled me away. I kept waiting for my husband to be allowed in, but they didn't let him. My husband was very scared and sad about not being allowed in the OR.

I had a nurse who was a member of the congregation that my husband was a pastor at. She was upset with my husband for expressing his disappointment over not being allowed to watch our son be born. She left the church shortly after. This has bothered me for a very long time. It felt like they were more concerned about their own feelings than ours. I had to go through the entire preparation and C-section alone. On top of it all, I was vomiting into a vacuuming tube they gave me to hold because they didn't have enough personnel to help. My husband missed the birth of his son because the hospital insisted they needed a nurse for each of us. This wasn't even an emergency, and my baby was doing just fine. Labor stalled, and they just wanted to get it over with.

After the delivery, they took him to the nursery, where my husband and kids got to watch him get cleaned up and hold him before me. This was my last baby, and I felt like I wasn't able to bond with him as well as with my other two. Having a C-section was so much harder than having two natural births. I think women who are willing to go through that again are very brave! I'm not sure I could do it again.

The vulnerability and lack of control over my own body, along with being scared to death going through it alone, left me sad and feeling robbed of the joy bringing new life into the world should have. My husband used to want one more child, but I knew I wouldn't because I thought my next birth would have to be another C-section. I think he wanted another baby because he didn't get to see our last son be born. Sometimes fathers are overlooked because the focus is on the mother and child. This experience affected him just as much as it did me.

I Wasn't Allowed to Meet My Babies

I ended up giving birth to twins vaginally in a huge public teaching hospital in Nice, France. I was forced under unconsented general anesthesia after having an epidural at 10 cm (which worked fine). They literally tied my legs down and restrained my body in restraints. It was truly barbaric! I had pushed out my first baby's legs, and then they forced the anesthesia mask over my face. There was no consent. I woke up, and the doctors were stitching me from an unconsented episiotomy. My babies were gone. I wasn't allowed to meet them, even though they were born in perfect health at 35 weeks. I was completely traumatized. Had I had proper coaching, support and had the hospital not strapped me in physical restraints, my cervix would never have begun to close on my baby's head. I had a vaginal breech birth with typical breech maneuvers, but at the expense of a huge trauma, as well as sadness for not being allowed to even see or meet my babies for 7 ½ hours after they were born.

Terrified That I Wouldn't Heal

Even though I had made the decision to try for a VBA2C, I never actually expected to succeed. Having two back-to-back failure to progress C-sections had completely crushed my confidence, and I truly thought my body was broken. When it finally worked, I was shocked. It was amazing…healing...freeing. Those feelings are still with me five years later.

But I knew within a couple of hours that something was wrong. This was my third epidural, and I was accustomed to what normal felt like. This was not normal. My right lower leg was completely dead. I could not flex my foot up or down. I informed the staff, but they told me it could take up to 24 hours to regain sensation. I decided to give them that long, but I knew the numbness wasn't going to go away.

They finally listened to me. I couldn't walk. I couldn't pee. I had to have a Foley catheter reinserted to drain my bladder because although I could feel the urge to pee... I couldn't actually do it. It was terrible.

When the 24 hour mark came, they decided to start evaluating me for underlying causes. The main concern for them was a spinal hematoma caused by the epidural. I was sent for an MRI of my spine and that was ruled out. At that point, they hypothesized that I had sustained some type of nerve damage.

My OB was out of town during all of this (she had a vacation planned the day after I gave birth). I was having to deal with doctors and nurses I had no relationship with, and that was difficult. They did not have any answers for me. I was told it could take six weeks to one year to regain sensation in my lower extremity. That was all the information I got. I had to advocate for myself and ask for a walker and a physical therapy consultation. The medical staff truly did not know what to do with me.

I was frustrated and scared by this. In my mind, medical professionals always knew the answer. I had always viewed them like House or Grey's Anatomy -- always digging for answers when they didn't know the answer to something. Unfortunately, this was not the experience I had, and I was so disappointed. It's the first time I ever saw that medical professionals are human, just like everyone else. They don't know everything. They make mistakes. And not all of them are willing to exhaust themselves to find answers for you because they are stretched thin and tired themselves.

People make fun of "Dr. Google," but it saved me in this experience. It gave me a name for my injury (peroneal nerve damage with foot drop) and connected me with a community of mothers on Facebook who had sustained the same, or similar, injuries. The group is called Moms with Femoral/ Peroneal/ Sciatic Nerve Damage from Labor/ Delivery.

This nerve damage is associated with lithotomy position and being in any hyperflexed position for too long during labor. It's important, (especially if you have an epidural) to make sure you are changing positions frequently while laboring. If you end up using the lithotomy position, make sure your medical team does not press your legs against the stirrups, as this cuts off blood supply to the nerves in your lower extremities. Women with epidurals are more likely to sustain this type of injury because they can't feel the damage as it's taking place.

It gradually started improving, starting at four weeks postpartum. That's the first time I could move anything. It was the slightest wiggle of my pinky toe. From then until ten weeks, I regained more and more sensation each day. At ten weeks, I had no remaining numbness at all.

I was terrified that I wouldn't heal. When the doctors and nurses couldn't really give me any answers, it felt like I was tossed into the sea, left clinging to a small glimmer of hope that I "might" recover. I wasn't confident in their time frame since they didn't even know how to adequately care for me. They didn't offer a walker, brace, etc., I had to request those things. It was obvious they hadn't dealt with many like me, so my confidence in them was shaken, and I couldn't trust their assurance that I would recover.

The moms in my Facebook group assured me that I would, though. They recommended all sorts of things from physical therapy to nerve exercises. I would scroll and scroll through the group, reading progress stories from other moms. That kept me hanging on, until it was my turn to post my own progress story.

NICU Experiences

The NICU provides care for premature and sick babies. Parents who experience the NICU have unique feelings surrounding it. It can be a roller coaster of emotion, ranging from gratitude, fear, grief, and more. Some parents are told during their pregnancy that their babies will likely go to the NICU, while other times it is a complete shock after delivery. Some parents have PTSD, or other lasting effects after these experiences, which requires support from those around them. Being thrust into the NICU makes you realize an inner strength that you never knew you had.

Don't Be Afraid

My twin girls were 5 weeks early and breech, so I ended up with a C-section. We spent 12 and 18 days in the NICU with them. Although the NICU seems very scary, it was honestly the best care we could have gotten. They know exactly what to do for your baby. Don't be afraid; they are there more than you know to help you and the baby. I would say all the nurses were phenomenal. The doctors were phenomenal, too! Our 18 day NICU baby was having trouble eating on her own, and they assured us with her being early, it was completely normal. Their brains just need more time to rest.

I Felt Like I Failed

My son was in the NICU for two weeks after his birth. He was born at 34 weeks. I was put on magnesium during labor, and I wasn't allowed to see my son for 24-48 hours because I wasn't allowed to walk and "needed to rest." It was heartbreaking. I had a C-section, and the moment he was out I couldn't see him, only through photos.

When I finally did see him, I was crying immensely. I hated to see him in the little box. I felt like I failed. I felt like it was all my fault. It really sucks when you're limited and can only show your new baby through photos.

They're not trying to be mean, and they're not trying to limit your rights. They're protecting every single baby in that NICU with low immune systems who can't fight off infections like we can.

I Was Not Prepared

My pregnancy was perfect. On the morning of 37 weeks 6 days, I woke up thinking I was having Braxton Hicks contractions. They kept getting stronger when I was at work, so I decided to call my boss and get a replacement. I called my husband and he took me to the hospital to be checked out. I was 4 cm dilated with contractions every 4 minutes, so they kept me for observation. In the afternoon, even though the hospital doesn't allow VBACs, they checked my cervix. Once again, like my previous two pregnancies, I was only 4 cm dilated. The surgical team was ready for the C-section. All my ultrasounds were perfect. There were no issues with the pregnancy. C-section prep went well until I laid down. The anesthesia was causing blood pressure issues. This has been something that got worse with each C-section, and they were unsure of the reasoning. The anesthesiologist gave me medications to keep my blood pressure up. Once stabilized, my husband was able to join me. Everything went well with getting to the baby.

My baby was delivered, and the staff went quiet. There was no baby crying. I started crying and hollering, trying to see what was going on, but unable to move. I knew something was wrong. I tried to talk my husband into looking over the sheet, but he wouldn't because he didn't want to see me cut open. The doctor said there is a complication and they needed to work on the baby for a little bit. My doctor started closing my incision. After what seemed to be at least an hour (not sure how long it really was), they finally let me see my baby. He was swaddled, not crying, and the longer he was by me, the more the purple color was increasing in his face. I instructed staff to take him back and do what they could. He was taken upstairs with his physician and nurses. My husband went with them, but I went to our room while they worked with our baby. It was the longest time I have ever had in my life, waiting in recovery to see if our baby was alive upstairs or what was even going on with him.

I was in my hospital room for a little while. They brought our baby in. He was in a warmer. Respiratory therapy had a mask over his face. Being a nurse I knew this was a ventilator mask. Occasionally they removed the mask and he started filling in with purple (cyanosis) and not breathing on his own. This was heartbreaking. I was at a local county hospital. The doctor said they usually wait a couple hours and sometimes they come out of it. She said little boys' lungs can be stubborn. I asked if he could be sent to a bigger hospital. They offered to send him to Des Moines. I did all my nursing clinicals in Omaha and knew a dash of comfort in this would be better. Children's hospital was offered, but I knew Methodist Women's would be my choice. During this process, they did stay in the room with my baby, working on him per my request. I knew he was going to be sent to a different hospital, so I took all the time I could get. To make it worse, I didn't know if I would ever see him again. The doctor came in and said the NICU will not allow ambulance transport and Life Flight was on their way. I had to sign financial papers, and that's when more stress set in. I had no idea if my health insurance covered Life Flight. My work health insurance is okay, but I have heard so many people paying on Life Flight until they die. I looked at my baby and knew he had to be taken anywhere to get help.

Black Hills Life flight arrived around 9:30 p.m. They took my baby and didn't come back for hours. My husband and I had work to do. We had to find people to take our other kids. I knew my husband was going to go with our baby to the city. We called his mom to go with him. I didn't want to have to worry about him driving over an hour, knowing our baby was flying in the air, sick or worse. Life Flight came in with a 10-15 foot long bed with a box my baby was in. Tubes were everywhere. IVs going. He only had a nasal cannula on at this time. I talked with Life Flight, and for infants they are able to ventilate a baby through a nasal cannula (high pressure air just through their nose). They had four staff to fly. The one end had about 8-10 oxygen tanks. Being a nursing home nurse, I knew one of our residents could make it to Omaha for an appointment and come back with one of these and still have some left. I asked ight Life Flight how many they thought he would need to get to Omaha. They guessed three tanks. They were frowning and wondering what kind of a question that was. I knew he was small and tiny. A grown human can make it there by car and back on one. I knew three, by helicopter, was not good. We signed more papers, and I had to say goodbye to my baby for what could have been the last time. To make it worse, I knew my husband had to go be with him. I was still paralyzed (well that's how it felt) from my C-section. I could hear the helicopter motors start. My husband sent me Snap Chats. We couldn't call because I was crying and I knew he had to drive.

Around 11:45 p.m. I looked around the room at what was a day I had played out in my head for over nine months. I had been so excited for my

89

other kids to meet our baby. In the past, family had come and visited. I looked around my room, and all there was left was my overnight bag on the counter across the room. There was no husband, no family, and worst of all no baby. Around 12:15 a.m. the doctor called from Women's Methodist to give me an update. They had completed X-rays and his lungs looked fully developed. They were going to run more tests and see what was going on. I called and updated my husband, as they weren't there yet. I was exhausted. I knew my baby was where he needed to be and my husband was with him. I woke up the next morning at 7:30. I was frantic. I hadn't heard anything and reality was still hitting me. I called my husband and he looked exhausted. Our baby was in a warmer. I could hear his very faint cry and he was squirming, but no one was allowed to touch him or comfort him. I know it was best for him, but that was so heartbreaking. My husband and mother-in-law stayed in the NICU with him while I was still in the hospital an hour away. I would get calls at least two times, up to four times a day. I would FaceTime in for doctor rounds so I could hear what they were saying. They ended up giving him Surfactant, which is for underdeveloped lungs, after two days because he continued to drop oxygen levels. They also allowed skin to skin with my husband. It was amazing. He said when they put our baby on his chest for skin to skin, his oxygen levels increased naturally.

My husband came and picked me up on day three. We couldn't drive fast enough. As soon as I walked in they asked if I was breastfeeding. I had been pumping in the hospital, but my milk was very minimal. They changed his diaper and weighed him. Then after I nursed him they would weigh him again and see how many ounces of milk he had drunk. This, to me, was amazing. I felt as if I was being graded, though. There was so much pressure. He had a feeding tube in his nose to supplement because of fatigue. We chose to have donated breast milk given to him until I had enough milk to feed him. It was great to have that option. Every day he kept improving and the ventilator was decreased. On day seven, it was removed completely! The ventilator said, "STOP VENTING."

All I could think was that this could have been horribly different. This may have been hard, but it was also amazing. The kids were able to come and visit. Anyone who wasn't potty trained was not allowed in the NICU. I needed them together! They wore undies to the room and then diapered so they didn't have an accident. They were only there for an hour. Then we had hospital lunch. My other kids were two and four years old. They didn't understand why they had to leave us again. That was stressful. We had amazing cousins in Omaha that let us take over their house so the kids were able to stay the night with us. Our parents and siblings were the best we could ever ask for. On day nine we were released with no follow up or further treatments. He is now a year and a half old, with no health issues. I was so scared when we tested positive for COVID, but he made it right through.

I know we are strong, but every once in a while we get a reminder of how perfect everyday life is. I took the other deliveries for granted. I was sad because my body wasn't able to have natural births, but I will never complain of this again. Either way kids are born, as long as they are healthy, is really all that matters.

For anyone else going through this, pray. Don't forget to take care of yourself. At first when we were in the NICU, I would think to myself, "Some of these kids haven't had parents visit for days." The longer we were there, the more I realized why. The NICU is constant alarms, medical staff coding, stabilizing, tube feeds, judging levels, and IVs. Walking around, the windows say how long the babies have been there. Some are there for six months up to twelve months. After day seven we had to leave. We had the other kids over night. We went out to supper, and it was so much easier knowing he was improving and the staff was incredible. The night nurse at the hospital sat with me the first night. We talked until I fell asleep. It sounds dumb, but I was not prepared. I often wonder if I knew there was a likeliness for complications, would that be easier?

I Didn't Know Which Baby Was Mine

My son inhaled meconium as a result of medical incompetence -- I was forced to keep him for an hour while waiting for the OB. As a result, he was in the NICU for 8 days for low oxygen levels. It was so hard. He was my first baby and I had no idea how to handle it. I was scared and angry because I felt like none of the staff listened to my concerns. They bathed and fed my son without asking me, and I had to fight to be able to breastfeed. I had to sit on a hard chair next to him instead of recovering how I should have. I had over 200 stitches, so this was extremely painful.

After my son was born, he latched and nursed while I was stitched up. It wasn't until an hour after he was born that his low oxygen levels were noticed. Then he was whisked away from me, and I didn't know what had happened or where he was for almost 8 hours. It was terrifying. I looked in the NICU window and didn't even know which baby was mine. Then, when

I did finally get to see him, they acted like this would prevent me from breastfeeding. I had to fight very hard to breastfeed on demand. I was never given any information about what had happened and was treated poorly by the hospital staff. I hope I never go through that again.

Back and Forth

My second child had a stroke at birth and had over 100 seizures recorded in the NICU after that. She's doing better now at almost 3 months old, but December was rough to say the least. She was in the NICU for a month, so there was a lot of back and forth. Then I got COVID, so I wasn't allowed at the hospital for two weeks while they quarantined her. That was the hardest part of it all, not being able to see her while she screamed on the camera until staff could suit up to get in and help her. That sucked.

We Felt the Presence of Jesus

Our experience with the NICU is one filled with love, NICU transfers, surgeries, trauma, adrenaline, hope, shock, and death. Our sweet boy was born very quickly and unexpectedly at 33+1. He was my second VBAC baby, and I had been released from the hospital around 8:00 p.m., less than 24 hours prior to his birth. I was only dilated to 1 cm with no contractions, but I had been bleeding for a couple of days. As this was my third child, there wasn't much concern. Later that evening around midnight, I had one intense contraction that woke me from my sleep, but I was able to sleep the rest of the night. In the morning I started having contractions. I kept my provider in the loop and had an office visit planned with her that morning. The bleeding hadn't gotten better, however, I was still contracting irregularly. She checked my cervix dilation again and I was at 3 cm. She sent me to the hospital to be monitored. While there it was confirmed that I was in active labor and we would be welcoming a preemie into the world. We waited for an ambulance to arrive so I could be transferred to a hospital with a NICU and Maternal Fetal Medicine Doctors.

I had a hard time wrapping my mind around birthing a small baby vaginally but was reassured that I could. My baby came out with the tiniest, yet strongest cry. His Apgar score was an 8 and we even had a little skin to skin time. It was the most perfect outcome for the most unwanted and unexpected circumstance. We were told we had a "feeder grower" baby and should hopefully be heading home in a handful of weeks. That all changed when he was just a week old. I was up pumping around 1:00 a.m.

They had upped his feeds again that day, and after coming off of TPN again, I wanted to see if he was tolerating them well. When I called they had just sent him back to X-ray to check his feeding tube and his tummy for a possible perforation. I naively thought it was no big deal because he had some issues a couple days prior and nothing came of it, so I thought that this would be the same. Finally, about an hour later, I received a call back from the NICU saying that our baby was very sick and that he would need surgery.

My husband and I had a long, quiet 20 minute drive to the NICU after dropping off our middle child with family in the middle of the night. We arrived at the NICU to see a rhythmic commotion happening because of our baby. We got to his side to see his tummy was swollen and a green color from the perforation. The neonatologist would eventually call for insulin, as his blood sugars were insanely high for such a little guy. The transfer from this NICU to Children's NICU, where they would do surgery, took a long time, and they were both in the same city. From what I can remember through the shock and exhaustion, it was about 5-6 hours from the time we found out that he was sick until he was back for surgery. These were some of the longest hours of my life. In this exhaustion, during his surgery, a social worker came to share details about the NICU, Medicaid, and other various programs. While I absorbed some of that information, my husband and I were completely exhausted. The doctor came out shortly after this time and shared that his surgery went well and it would be likely that we wouldn't have any more complications, just healing and growing. His stomach perforation was caused by a malrotated bowel.

We lived in the fantasy that all would be well until 6 days later, when we discovered suddenly again that he would need another surgery. When his stomach had perforated, Candida was released and it turned into an infection that settled in his abdomen. Following those two surgeries, we had three more surgeries in 5 days, then 9. The final surgery was 6 days later, and we found out that the infection had taken over completely. His bowel, which before had only a few very minor perforations, now had five perforations. His stomach was completely ripped and his duodenum and colon were dying. Our baby's body was no longer compatible with life.

I received this news without my husband by my side because he was on his way into town. The surgeon held my hand as I tried to absorb this news. I asked if there was a different hospital that we could transfer to and change this dire outcome, but the answer unfortunately was no. Their suggestion was to cuddle our baby and call family in while we could. At this point my husband showed up and the surgeon explained everything again and then asked us permission to not operate on our baby, just replace his stomach patch. He would be on life support until it was time for him to enter into eternity with Jesus.

Even with this amount of trauma, of which I explained is only the very tip of the iceberg, we absolutely felt the presence of Jesus and the strength of the church surrounding us. It's hard to see that in the darkest of days, but it was there. I can't even begin to list the amount of blessings we received during that stay and even almost a year later.

It Is All a Blur

My first born was in the NICU for 5 days. She had trouble getting enough oxygen, and there was meconium during the birth. They feared she had aspirated some and had an infection from it. She was on oxygen and antibiotics and had more labs done than I can recall. As we were about to be released, she became jaundiced, so we stayed another day to do light therapy. When we went home, the doctors said we could act as if she hadn't even been in the NICU. She was healthy and would not have any lasting repercussions from her rough start. Because it was our first child, we had nothing else to compare to. It was exhausting and emotionally overwhelming.

I didn't realize how much it impacted me until I had another child that didn't require extra care. It was so much different. I sometimes still feel guilty for not spending more time holding her in the NICU. I was a new mom and so timid. I didn't know the rules or if I would hurt her by holding her while she was hooked up to so many tubes and monitors. I also had to triple feed, which took so much time. We would always go back to our own room in between to try to sleep for a bit. It was constant trips back to her NICU room every 2-3 hours. After a triple feed session, we only had 30-45 minutes to sleep before we did it all again. In retrospect, I wish I would have asked more questions and stood up for myself and my daughter more. I wish we had more skin to skin time and wonder if the lack of it damaged her in any way. I wish I was able to appreciate the staff and nurses more. After so many shift changes and so little sleep, it is all a blur.

So Many Unknowns

My youngest was in the NICU for 24 days. He was born two days before COVID hit, so we had rules changing daily. Even with all of the changes, the staff was amazing. It was different from my other births. It was scary at times because with his genetic condition there are so many unknowns. I wasn't used to having others care for my child.

Trust the staff and absorb as much information as you can from them. One of the nurses made an impact for us by always making time to peek in and spend time with our baby. She was so patient with his feeding issues, and you could tell she put extra time and effort in to help him.

Amazing Beginnings

Our twins were born at 26 weeks gestational age. They completed the remainder of what would have been my pregnancy in the NICU at Tacoma General Hospital, Tacoma, WA. I saw my daughters for the first time immediately after I was stitched up and wheeled into a viewing room. I was very drugged but lucid enough to see they were beautiful. They were very thin and red, due to the skin not being fully developed, and looked like tiny little people from internment camps who were starving. But I thought they were pretty. I was so happy to see them. I asked if they were okay, and while not much was said in the way of an actual response, I believed they would be.

The next morning after the drugs wore off, I got out of the bed, had my husband get a wheelchair to take me to the NICU wing, and found my girls. The walking was awkward as the C-section left an enormous scar that was obviously not healed. There I began my crash course of how prematurity was managed. I learned everything possible for a layperson to learn. I needed to understand what was happening to them, what the specialized team was doing for them, and how they were responding to it. This became my job for the next 24 weeks. Fear was suppressed, as my job was to ensure they survived their early start.

There were moments of anxiety, joy, elation, terror, pride... and the cycle continued. I would say it finally subsided, but that's parenthood. That cycle continues 27 years later. Our NICU team was the first reason we knew without a doubt all would be okay. They became our friends. I became a non-sanctioned part of their professional landscape. These people were almost cavalier about our daughters' survival. "Of course they'll be fine. They're just little, that's all." I fed on their energy, and they encouraged my optimism.

Be with the babies every day. Talk to the medical team and ask questions. The doctors and nurses in the highest level NICUs are highly specialized practitioners and are the most advanced in their fields. They truly do God's work. The more you understand, the better a partner in the process of their healing you can be. Someone once said, "Yes, all that learning would be a good distraction." She was as stupid as her comment. In life we must be active partners, not bystanders. This kind of survival is not accidental. It is intentional. Be tough and intelligent and strategic. Plan for their survival and for them to thrive as your children were intended.

I've laid out my story very briefly for my "Tag Team Terrorists," that's what my twins were from birth on. Their prematurity survival was highlighted by one medical event to another in the earliest days and years. First one surgery, then another, then a correction, and then two...This continued into toddlerhood. Eventually it subsided and they were just children, children who had "amazing" beginnings. This word is so overused it's hard to know amazing when we see it these days. But my husband and I lived it. And they did, too.

We've tried hard to live up to their amazing start by showing them amazing parts of the world and experiences. Sometimes we succeeded and sometimes we faltered, like parents do. We apologized and then went on. The twins are now talented, brilliant and very independent young women. They will push through all walls in their paths, just as they did in the beginning. As for me, the Mom, I never felt like I didn't give birth. I've got the scar to prove it! To this day, I don't get the arrogance and ignorance of women who claim that giving birth has to mean that a baby comes through the birth canal. They need better education, which is entirely up to them. The avoidance of ignorance is a personal lifetime quest.

My Heart Broke for Those Babies

It was scary. All the wires, cords and machines that kept beeping. Seeing all the rooms with tiny babies in them was sad. Some had been there for months, and some you never saw have a visitor. My heart broke for those babies. I wanted to snuggle them all. My advice to someone going through this is to pray! Talk to your baby. Touch your baby. Sing to your baby. I believe all of those things can help a baby get well. All the nurses were great. They understood how important it was to stay updated and the sadness of not being able to hold your baby whenever you wanted. Many would go out of their way to help you be close to your baby or offer words of encouragement.

Each Day Is a Gift

I had an instinct that something wasn't right during my pregnancy. I wanted an ultrasound before we traveled out west, but insurance would not pay for it. I actually got into an argument with my husband because I felt so uneasy. He finally agreed to pay for one out of pocket. Surprisingly, everything looked fine on the ultrasound. They even said there are four chambers to his heart. Unfortunately, they didn't see the wall was missing, the arteries were transposed, and his aorta was narrow. Ultrasounds weren't as good back then.

Delivery was fast. I only labored an hour, and they were still trying to put the IV in me when I was pushing. I was shocked when he came out because he was so big compared to my first born. I thought, "That's not my baby, that's a two month old!" He looked perfect and even scored a 9 out of 10 on the Apgar. But, within the hour he started to turn dark purple. That's when we knew something wasn't right. The doctor assured us that it was just a temporary condition called transient tachypnea and it would clear up with some blow by oxygen.

They tried to treat him for this condition for about 12 hours in our small town. We were wanting them to move us to a bigger hospital, so they sent us to Kearney. In Kearny we checked into a hotel while they were running tests. They thought it had something to do with his lungs. Everything they tried wasn't working, and my husband started pulling books off the shelf and asking them, "Could it be this? Could it be this?"

Finally, they decided to do an ultrasound of his heart and an echocardiogram. That's when they said his heart looked like swiss cheese! They were not going to be able to help him there. They needed to fly him to Children's Hospital in Omaha. My husband decided to baptize him with a Dixie cup before he got on the plane. The reason why they used a plane instead of a helicopter is because my husband had just done a funeral for a nurse who died in a helicopter crash while transporting a patient, so we asked if they could take him by plane. A very nice nurse took a picture of our son with a Polaroid for me because we could not go with him. We were in the middle of a snowstorm, and we had to drive three and a half hours to get there. We beat the plane.

Once in Omaha we were not able to see him. The waiting room in the NICU was packed, and we were sitting in chairs in the hallway with other people. It wasn't until 3:30 in the morning, when he was a little over 48 hours old, that two doctors came out to tell us what was wrong. They showed us a picture of what a normal heart looks like and what my son's heart looked like, and they looked nothing alike.

He had three major problems, all fatal without medical intervention. They diagnosed him as having a rare heart condition called hypoplastic right heart syndrome. On top of that, he had transposition of the great arteries, so his aorta and pulmonary artery weren't going where they should go. He also had coarctation of the aorta, which means his aorta was narrow. The only thing keeping him alive at this point was the patent ductus arteriosus valve (PDA), which is a small hole in the heart of babies that allows blood to skip circulation to the lungs and closes soon after birth.

The doctors said we had three options. We could wait for a heart transplant, which would be 80% fatal because newborn hearts are hard to find, and he may not live long enough to get one. We could opt to do a surgery that had only been around less than 10 years and would give him a 50% chance of survival. In fact, they did the surgery on three children just the week before, and all three died. Or, since this was so bad, we could opt to take him home and let him die when his PDA valve closed, which would be anywhere from a week to a couple of months. We were told there was no wrong decision. They told us to take our time to decide over the weekend.

I fell apart and sobbed right there in the hallway among all of the other parents worrying for their own babies. I was overwhelmed with fear, doom and exhaustion. We were finally able to go see him in the NICU and pick him up to hold him. We were told he would probably need to be put on a ventilator, but looking at him in the NICU, he was the biggest and healthiest looking baby there. I couldn't help thinking how could he possibly be so sick? Despite looking so good, they said he was the most critical. After talking to my husband, we chose the only option that I thought would give our baby his best odds. We decided to have them do surgery on him.

He had three major open heart surgeries and other minor procedures. His first one was done when he was one week old on a Monday. They prepared us ahead of time by letting us see another baby that had surgery a few days before. The reason they did this is because with the first surgery there is so much swelling in the chest that they cannot close it back up. They left the baby's chest open, exposing the heart and lungs.

It was so hard to see the baby with his heart and lungs exposed, knowing that my child was going to be cut open the same way. I had an overwhelming sense of compassion for what that mother was going through, sitting next to her baby, not being able to hold him, hooked up to all kinds of monitors and IVs.

I spent every waking moment at my son's side that week, only going back to the Rainbow House, where we were staying, when the nurses made us leave at night. I cried and prayed constantly. I was haunted by hearing imaginary baby cries when I was alone. Thankfully, my son never had to be put on the ventilator, and I was able to hold him for that entire week, soaking him in, in case that was the only time we would have with him.

His first surgery took 12 hours. The reason why it has such a low survival rate is because they literally chill the body down so that the baby is lifeless while they build a new aorta. They make the right ventricle pump blood to the body through the new aorta. This is called the Norwood Procedure. It is also risky because it's very hard to restart a single ventricle heart. So my son was "dead" for 57 minutes while they worked. When they were done, he was hooked up to so many IVs, monitors, and machines, including a ventilator, and his chest was open. I was able to see his heart and lungs moving underneath a clear Gore-Tex patch that they sewed over his opening. Strangely it was not grotesque but very comforting to watch because it meant he was alive.

The NICU nurses were amazing and so were his doctors. His doctor would even call from home to check on him. The nurses even made a little tuxedo top out of a dinner napkin to place over his heart and lungs so that we didn't always have to stare at his chest.

On that Friday, they took him back into surgery to close up his chest. After a while, the doctor came back out to tell us he had good news and bad news. The good news was that our son was stable and doing fine. The bad news was they were not able to close his chest because he was still so swollen. They had never had that happen before. That was very unsettling and nerve-racking because we wondered what happens if you can't get his chest closed. They reassured us that they would try again in a few days. On that Monday they were finally able to close him up.

I was so grateful that we were able to bring our son home, but I was also terrified at the same time. While we were in the hospital they were keeping him alive, and we were told that he could die at any moment even after the surgery. I desperately wanted things to feel as normal as possible and to enjoy every moment with him. Knowing that we had to go through this at least two more times was devastating. He needed his second heart surgery at six months old because he outgrew the shunt they put in. I hated knowing that I had to bring my baby back in to be cut open, but it was his only chance of survival. I probably went overboard creating as many memories as possible for him and our family.

It was very hard during this time to pretend that I was okay and to keep a positive outlook while I was falling apart inside. It was especially hard as a pastor's family because you're supposed to show that you have unwavering faith in God, and even though I knew what would happen was God's will, I prayed without ceasing that He would let him live. I also had a lot of guilt for devoting so much time and energy to my baby when I also had a five-year-old at home. I felt I wasn't giving her enough attention.

Sometimes I wish that my present self could go back in time and tell my past self what God had in store for us. It has been 25 years. Most of his childhood I tried to let him be like any other child and never used his heart condition as an excuse to not be able to do something. We lived knowing that he could die at any time, that his heart might just stop working and there would be nothing we could do, even with the heart surgeries. His surgeries were so new back then that they never had children make it out of adolescence. Now they are reaching adulthood. He had his last major surgery when he was 2 ½ years old. Back then he thought that the crane fixed his heart because there was a giant crane working on building the new wing of the Children's Hospital. He has always had an innocent tender heart.

The doctors have told us that he is their best case scenario to date, and he is so lucky that he does not have to take any heart medications. God granted us a miracle on multiple levels. He allowed us to keep our son and watch him grow, but he also taught us how important it is to keep our family as a priority, to love each other fiercely, and to see each day as a gift. My son is 25 now, and although he may not be able to keep up with the fittest 25 year olds, for someone with his heart condition, he is doing great. Looking at him you would never know that he wasn't like everyone else.

Grief and Loss

Grief and loss take many forms and can be caused by many different things. We experience loss through miscarriage, stillbirth, adoption and even infertility. There are times we may not know how to support someone going through a loss. There are no magic words to make it all better. Sometimes the best thing we can do is say, "I'm so sorry for your loss. I'm here for you." We can offer a listening ear and sit quietly with their grief.

My Two Losses

When my husband and I were first married, we started trying right away. We got pregnant the first time we tried, and we were over the moon excited! I remember one afternoon when I was around 6 weeks pregnant, I took my dogs outside. When we walked back inside, I felt a "pop" in my pelvic area and the pain brought me to my knees. I couldn't walk for about five minutes. To this day, I still don't know what it was. I had no bleeding or anything following that, so I carried on like normal.

At my 8 week appointment they told me my baby looked to be falling behind in growth and to come back in two weeks to rescan because maybe our dates were off for conception. But I knew they were correct. We went to the 10 week scan to check on our baby, and they told me there was no heartbeat. My husband and I were crushed and cried from the hospital to our car. We sat there and bawled for the next hour. The doctor gave me cytotec to induce delivery of our angel baby. So I went home and inserted the pills the next day and waited. I had contractions for about 12 hours and delivered our baby at 10 weeks 2 days by myself on the floor of our bathroom while my husband was at work. We waited three months and got pregnant again. This was the pregnancy of our first born child.

Our second loss was easier for my husband than myself. When I found out that I was pregnant again, I was so excited, but my husband was a lot more cautious. We ended up losing that baby at 6 weeks along. It was very painful and just awful, but he acted like everything was okay. We tried for over a year to get pregnant again before finding out I was finally pregnant with our second born baby.

It Was Very Difficult

I was on Clomid for one month to get pregnant with my first daughter. I had bloodwork and ultrasounds every other day. There were injections and invasive testing. My first pregnancy ended in miscarriage at 14 weeks. It was a girl. I caught her in my hands. It was very difficult having a miscarriage. Then, when I couldn't get pregnant, I blamed myself.

Do what you feel you can handle, but don't give up because I was told I could only get pregnant with help, and I got pregnant on my own 14 years after my first daughter. Be kind to yourself and take whatever time you need to go through miscarriage or infertility. It is rough on our bodies!

It's Okay to Grieve

After losing my first baby right at the end, I was so worried during subsequent pregnancies that it would happen again. Carrying a child was exciting but terrifying, knowing I could come home empty handed. Even now, after four more healthy kids, we grieve on her birthday. When I hear someone I know is close to birth or going into labor, I pray hard and get anxious.

It's okay to grieve. Take your time to heal and pull close to God. Let your spouse grieve however they need to, even if it looks like they aren't at all. And while it's helpful to talk to others who have miscarried, don't ever compare losses, thinking yours was worse or not as bad as someone else's.

I Held Her in My Hand

Our miscarriage resulted in a heightened awareness of loss in the pregnancy that immediately followed our early loss. Once we were in the "safe zone" of 24 weeks, I thought that meant we would bring our rainbow baby home, a term I happily once used. Our rainbow baby was born at 33 weeks 1 day. We had a very traumatic NICU experience that ended just over a month later.

Our rainbow baby died. I realized there is no safe zone, and I cringe at the term now because not all rainbow babies come home. These back to back losses have obviously been very difficult for our family, but we acknowledge our grief. We acknowledge that God knows each of our days and that He will also carry us through in our darkest days. It has made me realize just how little control we truly have, and that can be hard to accept.

During our early miscarriage at 6 weeks gestation, I remember going to the bathroom at my midwife's office. I wiped and there was the very obvious baby and sac. It looked just like the pictures do at 6 weeks. I held her in my hand, hardly believing that it was actually my baby. I said, "I love you my sweet baby," and then I flushed. That moment was very odd because I am my children's protector, but it also gave me a sense of healing because I could tell her I loved her. I will forever remember that moment. We named that sweet baby Hope.

After our miscarriage and infant loss, I learned it's okay to have solid boundaries. To say yes to help, and that some days you just have to get that frozen pizza from the store… again. It's okay. Sometimes this is how we have to take care of ourselves to keep moving forward in a healthy way.

Our Individual Grieving Experiences

My first pregnancy was a miscarriage at about 6-7 weeks. I had already told family, friends, and coworkers that we were expecting because we were so excited we couldn't contain it. It was devastating to have to tell everyone we lost the baby. But I'm also glad these people knew because they supported us and loved us so well through it. We waited three months to try again and got pregnant right away and had a healthy pregnancy and birth.

My miscarriage was one of the most difficult things in my life. It was heartbreaking and so hard to explain to others. It made me worry a lot during my next pregnancy. We never named the baby we lost because it was so early on. Part of me felt bad about that at first, but I don't any more. I don't really think about it very often anymore, especially with two beautiful kids to keep me busy.

My husband experienced the loss in a much different way. I think it was because the pregnancy was not tangible to him yet. He hadn't felt the baby kick or experienced any of the pregnancy symptoms, so it was less real to him. Although I assured him that it was gone after I had bled so much, he needed medical confirmation that it was a true miscarriage. I knew, but he couldn't accept it until speaking with our midwife. It hurt me at the time. It felt kind of like a twist of the dagger that was already in my heart. I've learned that our individual grieving experiences are so much different. Just

103

because he processed it differently, doesn't mean he didn't feel it, too. Give your husband and yourself grace to grieve in your own ways, and be honest with each other through the whole process.

I found the most solace in talking with other women who had also experienced it. It was so hard to express my feelings over something so intangible with someone who hadn't also been through it. Statistics are so high for those who have experienced it. Don't be afraid to seek out a friend or acquaintance who has been through it, too.

Give Them Space

My miscarriages have impacted my health, well being, emotions, everything. It is so devastating to find out that you are pregnant and get it all ripped away within days or weeks. The excitement to know you are welcoming a baby into this world is ripped from your hands. It really takes a toll physically and emotionally. I remember crying and losing myself for the longest time. That pain, those feelings, they don't go away. It does get somewhat better over time, when you start accepting, but it's still that pain anytime the dates pass, etc.

If there is someone going through a miscarriage, they are probably not going to want to talk right away. Give them their time. Give them their space. Everyone reacts differently. We're angry, mad, sad and upset.

You're Not Alone

After my firstborn, I got Nexplanon in my arm. I had it for a year and took it out shortly after his first birthday. We struggled for 2 ½ years and had two early miscarriages. We saw a fertility clinic before getting pregnant with my second. I've had three total losses. All were early. The first two were only two months apart and similar. I got an early positive and started bleeding within a week after. My third miscarriage was the month before I got pregnant with my current pregnancy. I didn't test, but I was almost a week late. I was going to take a test the next day, but I started bleeding.

These miscarriages were some of the most painful things both emotionally and physically. It made me appreciate what I have. I was lucky to get pregnant while I was on birth control the first time. It truly is amazing that babies grow and are healthy the majority of the time, because so many things can go wrong. You're not alone. It can feel like your world is crumbling and that no one cares, except you, that you are losing a baby.

Or maybe you just can't get/stay pregnant, but there are women all over the world fighting similar battles as you.

Grief from Infertility

I was diagnosed with unexplained infertility almost nine years ago. It's still unexplained, and I'm still without a child to this day. My experience with infertility has greatly impacted every portion of my life. Aside from the effects of trying every medication and treatment available, there's the effects of the "maybes" and the "what ifs". "Maybe I'll be pregnant during such and such time, so I shouldn't book that vacation, just in case." While house shopping, "What if we do get pregnant? We need a house big enough to accommodate children." Along with the "what ifs," there is, "What if I caused this somehow? What if I could have done something differently? What if all this effort and all these years never pay off and I never become a mother?" What if, what if, what if? They constantly run through my mind with every possible question and possible outcome.

Infertility has mentally destroyed me. I suffer from severe chronic depression and anxiety, which of course has only increased due to the stress that accompanies infertility, as well as having ADHD and severe insomnia. I do not take any medications for these illnesses, as they're not proven to be safe for pregnancy, and I refuse to risk harming a baby in case I get pregnant. Infertility has also affected life-long friendships that are now non-existent due to the effects. Infertility has made me feel incredibly alone, as I'm surrounded by people with children and constantly see pregnancy announcements on social media. It seems like everyone, except me, is able to do the one thing I want more than anything. It's also incredibly infuriating to see so many people who make terrible parents have child after child. Infertility has a way of affecting your entire life rather than just being a part of it.

I would tell someone who's dealing with infertility, don't be ashamed. This is an illness, the same as diabetes or cancer. This does not make you inadequate as a woman. You have no control over it. Tell anyone who tells you, "Everything happens for a reason," where to shove it. There is no reason this has happened to you. Take all well meaning advice with a grain of salt, and ignore as much of it as you'd like. Join support groups on Facebook. It's so nice to be able to speak to people who actually get it, instead of people who just say to stop trying and it'll happen. Even if you choose to stay silent in the groups, just being able to read all of the posts is therapeutic. Don't be afraid to get a second opinion for anything. Sometimes a new set of eyes can catch something previous doctors have missed.

Grief with Adoption

I was scared to death when I found out I was pregnant. I was 16, and I had a hard time dealing with the unknown. My mom got pregnant 3 months after I did. Then my boyfriend cheated on me. When I was 7 months along, my dad told me I had to give the baby up because they were having one of their own and wouldn't have room for mine, too. I was also told if I didn't give her up, I couldn't come home.

It was a semi- open adoption. I asked for pictures and a letter until she was 18. They stopped all contact when she was 7. Legally there was nothing I could do. It impacted my relationship with my parents. It definitely impacted how I parent my own kids and being very overprotective to the point it isn't healthy. Adoption grief and trauma therapy helped so much. I finally realized I needed some help at age 35, seven years ago.

Being pregnant as a teenager isn't something any parent wants for their child. When your kids tell you something, don't blow up or freak out. Speak calmly to them. Have open and honest conversations with your kids about sex, teen pregnancy and STDs. I've learned not to react like my parents did, and my relationship with my kids is very open. Sometimes I hear things I don't want to hear. Sometimes my kids get in trouble, but I'm not unreasonable, and I explain why they're being disciplined for an action or behavior. I can proudly say my oldest child didn't have sex until 18 and my 15 year old is still a virgin. With the other two, that's a way off yet. My oldest two have both told me they waited because of how honest I was, and still am, with them. Communication makes a difference, and the way you communicate makes an even bigger difference.

Be Patient with Yourself

I was five months along when I lost my third baby. Apparently he stopped growing weeks before. My doctor told me that I could go home and would probably start to cramp and pass the baby in a few hours.

We were stunned. My husband and I went home and waited, but I didn't feel anything until around 1:00 a.m. I started to have contractions and started to bleed. I had contractions all night long. I passed large blood clots the size of my hand, each time wondering if it was my baby. I labored all night in the bathroom, getting weaker and weaker until my baby came out in the toilet at around 11:00 a.m. the next day. I quickly picked him up out of the blood clots and held him in my hand.

He was perfectly formed, and I could tell he was a boy. He had tiny fingernails and fit in the palm of my hand. I cleaned him and talked to him. My husband baptized him. We put him in the plastic container the doctor provided me so we could bring him back and have genetic testing done and then have him cremated.

By the time I delivered my baby I had lost so much blood, and was so dizzy and weak, I could hardly get up off the floor. My husband took me to the hospital. I was freezing and could not control my shivering. They gave me an IV with fluid and said I had lost two units of blood. My doctor came in smiling at me and said she was surprised that he came out in one piece. Then she sent me home. I was devastated, exhausted, and crying uncontrollably. I did not feel right.

Soon after I got home I started having contractions again. I felt like there was something else inside me, and I felt a bulge, but I didn't know what it was. I was terrified, not sure if it was a blood clot. If I pulled it out, would I bleed to death? I quickly called the hospital to talk to a nurse and asked her if I should try to pull whatever it was out. She told me not to, but to quickly come back to the hospital.

I could barely sit up as my husband drove me back to the hospital. Once we were there, a doctor examined me and realized that I had not passed the placenta. He was furious that they had sent me home to have my baby. He set me up in a hospital room and had me lay on the bed and helped me deliver the placenta. I was hospitalized for the night. It was such a long night. I never felt so alone, having to hear babies crying.

Since we were not sure why our baby died in the womb, and we already have a son with a genetic defect, we sent the baby away for genetic testing to find out if we should try again. We got his ashes back and visited with a genetic specialist who told us that he had Trisomy 18 (Edward's Syndrome). We were told that babies with this condition normally miscarry very early on and very rarely go this far or to term alive. If they do make it full term, they usually pass away soon after birth or within the first year.

After I came home, so many women came to the house to visit and bring food. Although I know they were all well meaning, I really did not want to hear their words of comfort. Some of them shared their own stories of miscarriage and cried with me, but some would give me advice that I did not want to hear. One woman told me, "You're going to want to try to have another baby, but another baby is not going to make it all better." Another woman actually asked me what my goals were now. All I could think of was to have another baby.

Honestly, I knew what I needed and what was best for me. What was best for me was to try and have a baby in my arms. We all grieve in different ways and need different things. It's very important to not judge each other for how we grieve. Grieve as long as you need, and be patient with yourself and forgive yourself. Allow yourself to feel what you feel and know that no feelings are wrong.

As heartbreaking and gut wrenching as it was to lose my son, we were told that this was probably a fluke and go ahead and try again. Sometimes God takes our grief and turns it into blessings because if we would have never gotten pregnant with him, we would've never decided to try for another baby. Although another baby could never replace him, our rainbow baby boy was born exactly a year later, on the very day that we were told our baby had died.

I Became Obsessed

My husband and I tried for about a year and a half to get pregnant. We were getting ready to look into our next options and see a fertility specialist. I found out in December 2019 that I was pregnant, and then I had a miscarriage a couple days after. I was very depressed. I felt like a failure, and sex was not fun anymore. I became upset when I saw friends on Facebook were pregnant and when I saw pregnant people out in public. I became obsessed with the idea of getting pregnant, and that made it harder each month when my period came. My advice would be to tell your partner/spouse exactly how you are feeling. Speak out about your miscarriage. I told only my parents, sister, and sister-in-law right away. I still haven't told a lot of people, but I found that with each person I told, a weight was lifted.

It's a Private Matter

I had one miscarriage/tubal pregnancy that terminated very early on. It was really just a fact of life for me. I know that a high percentage of pregnancies end, and I expected that I could be one of those who experienced it. What I wasn't aware of was how physically painful a miscarriage could be; the contractions were quite strong even that early on. I think that made me empathize with other mothers, especially those who experienced several and had the additional pain of heartbreak. I don't wish to be part of some "club" of women based on what I see as a normal biological event. I think that it is a private matter, and I don't like getting tagged in social meetings because I should identify as a... whatever it is that I am supposed to identify as. If you are going through this, it is not your fault. You don't deserve this. It's okay to mourn, and it's okay to be nonchalant.

Grief Is Not Once and Done

I've had four miscarriages, and three of them were within one year after the age of 40. With my last I had to have D&C. I had genetic tests to see if there might be a reason for miscarrying so many times (after already having four children prior to the age of 40). With the testing we found out it was a boy with Down's syndrome, but we were never really given an explanation whether or not that was why I had miscarried at almost 10 weeks. I had a D&C one year prior to this one, but no tests done, and then in between those two D&C's, I had a miscarriage that took over a month before I opted for the misoprotol pills. That took two separate doses, and I ended up miscarrying with heavy bleeding while out of town trying to help my sister pack and move. I had to tell her about the miscarriage, as she didn't know before that. So having three in one year was pretty depressing, and I only told a handful of people about any of it. It gets pretty lonely, and I feel lost as I'm always wondering why. I still haven't gotten pregnant since, and now I'm nearing 43, so I'm not sure there's any hope now.

Of the last three miscarriages in the last year (of four total -- the first being over 15 years ago), the hardest part was not telling many people and dealing with my emotions basically with very little outside support. The last miscarriage happened in May of 2020, right at the beginning of COVID, so I wasn't getting out much anyway and was working from home. I normally love the month of May, as it reminds me of new life with the start of spring, and my birthday and wedding anniversary are in May. School got out in May and my oldest daughter was set to graduate from high school on my birthday, May 17th. It ended up that I had the D&C just four days after Mother's Day. I found out there was no heartbeat two days before Mother's Day but had to wait almost a week for the procedure. This was three days before my birthday and the graduation day for my oldest daughter (although with COVID it was postponed to June).

My midwife hugged me and was so amazing, but the OB who did the procedure was more mechanical and not empathetic as I stared again at the perfectly formed fetus with no heartbeat on the ultrasound screen a second time to confirm what my midwife already knew -- that my baby was gone. I remember asking through a dumb mask, tears rolling down into my mask, "If you do the genetic tests, will you be able to tell me if it was a baby girl or a baby boy?" The non-empathetic doctor said in his medical terminology, "Yes, the test will tell if the fetus was a male or female." It was like somehow saying the words "baby boy" or "baby girl" would give it too much meaning, and he'd have to recognize that it was a real baby that had life but was now gone. I felt like him saying "male or female fetus" was so cold and clinical as I was trying not to sob into my bed sheet and mask.

I had a great experience with some other select staff at the hospital where the D&C was done. Even the admitting desk lady saw some alert on my chart and said, "I'm so sorry for your loss. I'm sure this is not easy for you," before getting down to business. For some reason someone just taking one minute to acknowledge my pain and loss of a baby meant so much to me. It was a simple gesture that only took 30 seconds of her time, but it meant a lot. They also provided me with a folder for parents who've lost babies at any stage, with resources and offers for burial of remains and baby memorial services. I didn't utilize this, but it was such a thoughtful thing that they had all this available. This last miscarriage I would have had the baby just two months before my sister had her last baby (also a boy), so they would have grown up together. Seeing her new baby son grow without seeing my own may be an ongoing loss, which I'm sure will hit me unexpectedly with grief and pain.

My advice for anyone going through this is to ask questions to find answers if that will help you heal. Don't stop until you find answers (if that will help you, if that would lead to more sadness and stress, then it's not necessary). Find someone, even if it's just one person, to confide in who will listen and not placate you, someone you can trust and who knows you well. Keep talking about it as you process the loss over time. Grief is not a once and done; it can hit at the strangest times. Take time off from work if you need to grieve. Explain to your boss as much or as little as you feel necessary. One wise pastor once told me, "You don't owe anyone an explanation. It's up to you how much or little information you share with any given person. Just because somebody asks does not mean you owe them any information."

I Felt Inadequate

I have PCOS. My first pregnancy was a surprise. The next time I tried to get pregnant, it wasn't as easy as I thought it would be. After a year of trying, we resorted to fertility pills, Clomid, and it took another six months to get pregnant again. I have had numerous miscarriages. Three were before 10 weeks and one at 14 weeks. The 14 week miscarriage was the hardest because in my mind, after 12 weeks you're supposed to be in the clear.

Trying to get pregnant was frustrating, and I felt inadequate. I had had an abortion between my first and second babies, and I worried that it ruined my uterus, or that not getting pregnant when I wanted to was my punishment. I didn't want to have an abortion, but I was a single mother and my partner was not the man I wanted to spend my life with. I was told by my parents that if I didn't marry him, I had to get an abortion or they would have nothing to do with me. I often wonder if when I die my lost babies will be waiting for me in heaven.

We Heal in Different Ways

I had a miscarriage at 20 weeks. I was 19, and the father wanted me to have an abortion. When I found out, I was already 17 weeks pregnant. I was scared and numb. I didn't tell anyone but the father that I call a "sperm donor" because he didn't want the baby. He harassed be for two weeks about getting an abortion, so I lied and said I miscarried to get him to leave me alone. Two days later I found out it was a boy. I started to wrap my head around it all. My sister was 20 when she had her first kid. If she can do it, I can too right? I went to bed that night with a whole plan to tell my family the next day, but that day never came.

I woke up in the middle of the night in terrible pain and bloody sheets. I went to a free clinic, and they Informed me I was having a miscarriage. They walked me through the whole process, and then at the end asked if I wanted to see/ hold him. I was in shock and so numb that I refused to see him. The clinic I went to didn't take good enough records to even find out why I lost my baby boy. I forced myself to act like I was never pregnant because no one else knew, so why tell them now? For six years I kept it a secret until the truth came out. It took me a few years after to feel comfortable to share my story with others when the topic came up. Sometimes I'm able to hide my emotions, while other times I break down.

I'm now 30, with a one year old and another on its way. There are still many who don't know I had a miscarriage, but I'm comfortable now sharing. The one thing I regret was not seeing him or holding him. To this day it still haunts me. I question if I jinxed it, if it was my fault somehow. I still don't know why it happened. When I share my story there are times it might seem I'm not very emotional, and that doesn't mean I'm not. It's been a few years for me, and I went through a lot to get to this point. Even though I'm strong enough now to hide the emotions, I still cry at times missing him. When I see my daughter play by herself it hurts knowing she could have had a brother with her to play. We all heal in different ways. Never feel ashamed for what you are feeling and know it's not your fault either.

I Appreciate the Children I Have

I got pregnant very easily. I would stop taking birth control, and my doctor would advise how long until I would be able to conceive. I was always pregnant before the window was up. I miscarried every other pregnancy early on. I appreciate the children I have a lot more than if they had come easily. I focus on the timing. I would have different kids if the other pregnancies had worked out. A lot of people tried to talk to me about loss. I would've rather done things with these people without talking about what had happened.

Allow Yourself to Mourn

I've had two miscarriages. My very first pregnancy ended in miscarriage, and then I had one after my second child. I was heartbroken with my first miscarriage. We had our first child about 18 months later. She wouldn't be here if I hadn't had a miscarriage, so I try to look at it that way. My second miscarriage was an unplanned pregnancy. We hadn't told many people I was even pregnant. I think the only person we told was my mother-in-law because my husband told her, and then she blabbed to more family. I was mad he told her because I wasn't ready for people to know. Then I miscarried and those people didn't know. It was very awkward when I had to tell them.

I would advise people who have miscarried to allow yourself to mourn if you need to mourn. It is a great loss. Allow others to mourn with you. It wasn't just your loss. For me, it always eases the pain to share the experience with someone you trust and love.

Motherhood Is a Journey

Being a Mother is a complicated thing. For me, just getting there was a bumpy road (pardon the pun). Not only does everyone experience pregnancy a little differently, each pregnancy is an entirely different experience in itself. I felt different about each pregnancy because of my age, maturity, and season of life. I have learned now to respond to a woman's news of pregnancy with a tentative, "How do you feel about that?" before offering ecstatic congratulations.

My first pregnancy came after four years of marriage. We felt like we were ready to start a family, and we were over the moon excited! Although I could hardly hold down ice chips for four days, and was sick often, I still felt like this was my time to shine. I marveled at every little kick inside me and talked to my daughter often. I was so sure that she and I were under God's special protection. That is why I struggled so much with my faith after we lost her.

My husband and I had a birth plan, and we had taken Lamaze classes together. We wanted it to be as natural as it could be. I was deathly afraid of surgery, and I was afraid if we were induced at all we would end up with a C-section. I thought I had communicated this to my doctor, but on that last checkup, after having lost my mucus plug, he stripped my membranes to "get labor going." I thought he was feeling for the head and position, and when I sat back up, it had been done. I was frustrated that he hadn't consulted me first. I went to bed that night with high hopes that we would have a baby in the morning.

I woke up exhausted, with a tight tummy and a low grade fever. I wasn't sure if the pressure was just part of labor or if something was wrong. I waited to go in, afraid of being pressured into a C-section. But by the afternoon she had stopped moving, and by the time I finally got a hold of my husband to drive me to the hospital it was 4:00 p.m. I had contractions on the way, 5 minutes apart. I remember the sunset was a brilliant pink; it was so beautiful we wanted to stop and take a photo, but there was no time. Looking back, I think it was the angels welcoming my daughter home.

They put a fetal monitor on, and after losing her heartbeat, rushed me into an emergency C-section. I counted down from 10 into a dreamless sleep while they took three minutes of desperate surgery slicing me open and pulling her out. When I woke up they had her in a box with a breathing tube. They told me to touch her. I couldn't understand what was happening. I got one touch over the glass and they whisked her away.

All night I cried and tried to sleep – alone, while my firstborn fought for life in a city 75 minutes away. They poked and prodded me and tried to figure out what had gone wrong. We called relatives, and my mother-in-law was flying out. When I heard this I threw down my hospital breakfast and yelled at the doctor that it was not fair for my mother-in-law to hold my baby before I got to. He quickly ordered an ambulance to come get me. He told me that our baby hadn't gotten enough oxygen and she was "very sick." He also said we would "have to make a difficult choice."

I felt every bump in the road in the ambulance as my pain meds wore off. The medic prayed for me. I bawled. When I finally got to Children's Hospital they housed me on the other side at an adjoining hospital and made me walk with my walker, in my butt cheeked gown and slippers, down the hall through a million buzzed in corridors to see her. She was almost 9 pounds, with beautiful long black curly hair. She didn't look sick at all compared to the other NICU babies. She just looked like she was sleeping. We held her as she slept. I never saw what color her eyes were. She was on life support, hanging lifeless with no brain activity for three days, while we, and the congregation we pastored, and the whole town, prayed hard for a miracle.

We had to talk to people who might want her organs for their baby, but we decided at the end not to take them. They said we would have to take them out while she was still on life support, and we couldn't agree to that, not if her miracle was coming. Even on that last day, as we stood beside her, watching her tubes come out, we hoped for the sound of a first breath or a cry. It never came.

Now, I don't do well with dead things. I didn't want to see my grandmother's open casket, and I really didn't want to hold a dead baby. But I let them take her to a little grieving room where all of the relatives that had come from far and near would get to pass her around. She looked like a tightly bundled doll, and her face was swelling and turning purple. I could hardly bring myself to touch her then. I felt so bad that I felt repulsed by this passage. Afterwards they told me that her heart was still beating for 30 minutes after they unplugged her. Then I had horrible guilt that I had asked them to take her away. I was glad that grandma had stayed with her until the end, even when I couldn't.

I cried out to God that night, not knowing if I would ever have children again. That night I had a dream that my daughter was an older girl, and she was a spirit, watching me buckle two little boys into the backseat of our car. I knew that it was a promise to me that in time, I would have two boys. It was a great comfort to my heart, even though I was disappointed in God for letting this happen. It seemed like He was there with me, not like the chaplain who wasn't even on duty the night we went to the chapel to plead for her life.

I shocked the chaplain when he came in to see me. I chastised him for not being there when we went to the chapel to pray. When he offered us plaster casts of her hands and feet, I thought he meant her handprint pressed into clay (like they do in kindergarten), but he returned with what looked like white chalky severed limbs from the Munster Show. I gasped and told him to get them away from me. He said, "I have never had a parent react like that before."

I went home empty handed, and deeply wounded, with full breasts and a swollen empty belly. There were so many people around trying to be helpful. Some people said, "You will have another baby," and, "When the going gets tough, the tough get going," and, "At least you aren't changing diapers right now."

There was nothing for me to do with my emptiness. There is nothing sadder than a quiet, dusty nursery. The funeral director asked if I wanted to choose a casket. There was NO WAY I was going to let her bring a baby casket into my house. I told her I'd take the cheapest one. It ended up being white and as small as a shoe box. We braved a funeral with the whole community, including my doctor, in attendance, and then we put the box in the ground.

Everyone grieves differently, and I had to go through the whole range of emotions. I wanted to grieve it thoroughly. It seemed so random and senseless. Later we found out that I had a common bacteria, Strep B, on my skin. Normally they give the baby antibiotics right after birth to counteract this. What they didn't know was that if you strip the membranes, it can pass bacteria into the baby's bloodstream.

I walked away from this experience knowing that if the doctor would have listened to my gut feelings about not having any kind of induction technique, my daughter might have been born a healthy 9 pound girl. I was so afraid of a C-section, and of being pressured into something, that I didn't go to the doctor right away, and I lost precious time where we could have saved her. I learned that I can tell a doctor "NO," and I can choose what happens with my body. There is really something to "mother's intuition" when it is balanced with doctor's advice.

The only way we survived this loss was believing that God is in control and all things work together for good. I knew my doctor would never make that mistake again, and he went on to deliver two more of my babies.

My husband and I grieved together. It was devastating, and we ended up leaving the ministry because we didn't have anything to offer needy parishioners when we had an empty cup. My husband got a science job, we adopted a puppy to cuddle, and we got pregnant again as soon as we could.

My second pregnancy was different. I was so happy, but so paranoid I'd lose him. Some mother's get past the time that they miscarried their last one and feel relieved, but because mine was lost at the last second, it was an entire 9 months of worry. I couldn't get him out soon enough. It was only 18 months after my C-section that we were having another. I didn't care how much weight I gained, or how we needed to get the baby out, I just wanted him to survive. At numerous doctors visits I would cry hearing the heartbeat (because that is all I ever heard from my first), and after telling them that I had lost one before this, the nurses would say, "Some people lose them before they even know they are pregnant." On the operating table, as they put the spinal tap in, I tried to hold in my fearful sobs as the nurse tried to comfort me by asking me gently if I had other children.

This time I was awake through it all, and I was so relieved to hear a cry at the end of it. We gave him a name meaning "Mighty Warrior" because we hoped he would fight to survive. But they wouldn't let me hold him. They stitched me up, and when I finally saw him, I almost fainted. He was lying with a plastic hood over his head. They said he wasn't breathing well and needed to be on oxygen. An alarm went off when I snuck him out of the hood to try to hold him, and they took him away from me. I was furious. The doctor left the room when they told me that they were going to send him to Children's in Omaha. At least this time they promised to send me too. It was another lonely, bumpy ambulance ride for me. (Don't those things have shocks?)

I was in trauma stress mode as I followed them down to the same NICU and saw THE SAME NURSE that had cared for my firstborn. Finally, eight hours after birth, I was allowed to walk down the buzzing corridors and hold my son. We got to do skin to skin, and I was so happy that he was alive! I walked it every two hours through the night to try to nurse him, which was difficult because I had to keep telling them not to give him a binky because it might mess up his ability to latch. We took him home in a huge blizzard at the end of February. Everything about his baby days was a struggle:

jaundice, nursing, sleeplessness… I was so stressed and tired that I could hardly hear any advice about what I was supposed to be doing.

I was paranoid that somehow I would lose him, and I worried constantly into his toddler years that tragedy, something I now knew I wasn't immune to, could always be around the corner.

Our second son was born two years later, with no complications, and no ambulances or helicopters. We gave him a name which means "Yahweh (God) brings healing." It was a beautiful thing, and I marveled at how quickly I healed from my surgery without the weight of trauma and sorrow.

Even so, my heart still longed for a daughter, for my first baby. We heard of a teenage pregnancy and offered to adopt the baby girl, but the mother kept her baby. God whispered to me that if we got pregnant again we would have our own girl. We did, two years later, and gave her the middle name Jubilee. Jubilee is a festival of freedom celebrated on the seventh set of seven years in Jewish culture. She was born seven years after we lost our first daughter, so it was our year of Jubilee.

At that point I was content to be done having children. My quiver was full, and I was glad to not have the worries of birth any more. We prayed to be done, but God had other plans. Even though He knows that I don't like surprises, not even surprise gifts.

Never mind how happy I should have been, I was upset when I discovered I was pregnant a fifth time. The doctor had warned me not to have too many C-sections, how dangerous it was, and I didn't want to go through it all again. Again, there was waiting and the sickness, and worry, with the diapers and sleepless nights, and exhaustion. Not to mention we then lived two hours from the nearest delivering hospital.

But I got used to the idea, and our third son arrived safe and sound. We gave him the name meaning "Gift of God". We were definitely ready to officially be done having babies. I had been cut open five times, so I let my husband do his part and get a vasectomy. It turns out that God knew I would need this little man to help comfort me in the rocky years of ministry ahead of me. God's plan is mysterious, but I wouldn't have it any other way.

My advice to new mothers struggling with feedings and schedules, and births and parenting is to let go of control. God's way is perfect, and He has His plans and his reasons. God opens and shuts the womb, and God heals the hearts of all the mothers who have been disappointed by how things turned out. These things are for a season, and it feels like the longest season ever sometimes. On those perfect summer days, when the toddlers are finally asleep or playing nicely, soak it in, the slowed down time, and hold that memory forever.

Motherhood is a journey, and it is said that each child is born into a "different" family because the dynamics change with each baby. For some it is blissful, for some a nightmare. It is always, always LIFE CHANGING

Postpartum and Breastfeeding

There are so many variations of normal when it comes to postpartum. To some, breastfeeding comes naturally, while for others it is a difficult, and sometimes even painful experience. Some parents bond with their babies instantly, while others take some time. Postpartum is a journey in itself, ranging from postpartum depression, breastfeeding challenges and re-discovering who you are.

I Wouldn't Change a Thing

I knew I had to at least try to breastfeed. I thought about how much cheaper it would be and how much more convenient, too. However, I didn't realize how utterly difficult it could be: chaffed/cracked nipples, bleeding, supply fluctuations and the judgment from so many people who are supposed to support you. But I wouldn't change a single thing. I was one of the first in my family to extend breastfeeding past a year (maybe even six months). I'm going to be on my third journey come June, and I'm more than just excited!

Breastfeeding Didn't Work Out

I was disappointed in my body. I dreamed of breastfeeding, and it just didn't work out. I have very flat/inverted nipples, and I tried everything I could to breastfeed. I latched him for three days before I switched to exclusively pumping. Once again my body failed me, and I was not producing any milk. I tried everything to get my supply up, but the more I pumped, the less milk I got until I wasn't getting anything at all. I had to hang up the pumps at four weeks postpartum.

Tongue Tie

Breastfeeding was very difficult with my first baby. She had a tongue tie that the hospital did not tell us about. We later had it clipped by our pediatrician, which helped a little. I had to do triple feeds in the hospital since she was in the NICU and my milk took a long time to come in. I was never a big producer throughout her first year, and I ended up exclusively pumping after about six months. I had a love/hate relationship with it, but mostly hate. I was just too stubborn to stop. It came so much easier with my second. My milk supply was more than we needed, and I was able to donate to some other moms in need.

Breastfeeding Wasn't for Me

I did not breastfeed. When I was 18, I thought it was gross because I didn't know anyone who had breastfed. This was in 1991. With my second baby, I had damage to the milk ducts in one breast from surgery, and so I didn't even try.

Indifferent

With my second daughter, I had postpartum depression. As sad as it was, I felt indifferent towards her.

More About Bonding

With my first, I felt pressured. I HAD to breastfeed because I couldn't afford not to. I made it 12 months, which is an accomplishment I was extremely proud of. Then with my second, I had to nurse because of money, but I was so over-tired, overworked and over-committed. It was just another task. With my third, I was frustrated. My first two breastfed so easily; I just assumed it would be that way again. My third baby struggled to latch, spit up a lot, and had a hard time gaining weight. I had to change my diet drastically and ended up supplementing early on, which led to supply loss and a real sense of failure. We made it eight months, mostly just comfort nursing. It was definitely more about bonding than it was about feeding. I also felt dismissed by the lactation staff at the hospital when they said things like, "Oh this is your third, you're an expert." This was NOT helpful!

I Should Have Asked for Help

With my first, I was lonely. I was all by myself all day, responsible for this amazing little life, how?! With my second, I felt anxious. I definitely struggled here and probably should have asked for help. It's hard to see it when you're in it. It felt like I had to do it all right now. When a visitor would come, I'd use the time to go scrub a bathroom or make pie or something not so important. I created things to keep me busy, and I stressed over these made up priorities.

With my third, I was disappointed. Our third child was born the day COVID shut the world down. My maternity leave was spent homeschooling my older children, which was far from the nap filled days of snuggling I had imagined.

Half the Battle

Postpartum hit me very hard. I didn't even realize what it was until my fourth child, who combined with an already hectic life, created a family of six! Knowing what it was, was half the battle for me. I also learned how important it was for me to find positive things to do.

Recovery Was Easy

I felt great. I had unmedicated births for both of my children so I was able to move around and recover pretty easily. My first was a little bit more difficult because I tore my clitoris in half. With my second, I was up and showering while they did all the baby's check ups. It was so nice to get all clean before settling in with my baby for the night.

A Stressful Experience

I had a hard time. As someone who's depressed, I didn't realize that postpartum depression would feel any different. I had about two people near me in my support system and lived 1,000 miles away from my entire family. It was terrifying. Breastfeeding was a struggle due to lip/tongue ties and a shortness in supply. We did therapy for the ties, but ultimately I tried to pump as much as I could since she wouldn't latch. That was a stressful experience all in itself once I realized I wasn't actually producing as much as she needed to eat. Breastfeeding lasted for just under two months.

I Felt Guilty

I think at first it was really hard for me. I kept having flashbacks of the C-section and just hated how it went. I remember being in the hospital having a dead look on my face and the nurses kept asking if I was okay. I remember just wanting to yell at them, "Yes, I'm fine, but I'm exhausted and just had my child ripped out of my stomach when neither he nor I were ready for it!" I felt embarrassed because they expected me to be so happy and cheery. I had maybe one hour of sleep that first night and the second day was even worse because they force you to walk around when you feel like your guts are falling out.

Then I felt guilty because my emotions weren't up to everyone's standards, but I knew how I felt on the inside and I loved my baby. I just don't think anyone understands, and I have always struggled with mental health, so I wasn't any different than normal. Overall I feel surprisingly fine. As I am typing this, I am three months postpartum, meaning I am three months into motherhood. Some days are a struggle, but it's worth it. At the beginning I was exhausted and overwhelmed, but everyone close to me said I adjusted very well. I'm still struggling to get sleep, but I think after a while you get used to it.

Different Each Time

I had no issues after my first, just general soreness and average exhaustion. With my second, however, postpartum depression and anxiety hit hard. I believe it was a result of a fairly traumatic delivery.

I Struggled

I struggled with the usual, like feeling beautiful and sane of mind. With my last one, though, I can truly say that was the only time I wanted to die. I struggled from an acute panic attack disorder that became chronic due to the drop in hormones my body had. I had lost an ovary due to cancer, and I also just had a baby. My body was all sorts of messed up. I couldn't breathe. It constantly felt like I was having a heart attack. Everytime I stood up, my blood pressure would drop, making me want to fall over. I couldn't walk, talk, sleep or eat. I could barely breastfeed my daughter. I was in this constant loop of panic attacks and I still struggle with it to this day almost 2 years later.

Postpartum Depression

With my first pregnancy, I was very calm and happy. With my second pregnancy I felt alone, sad, and once I tried to decide if I wanted to throw the baby down the stairs or out the second story window. I had postpartum depression.

We Never Looked Back

With my first son I got severe postpartum depression. My husband could not take time off to be with me and our son in the hospital. My son wasn't ever getting full and would just cry all the time. It was only later we found out I could not produce enough milk for him because my right breast had cysts throughout. I couldn't produce on that side and the other never produced more than an ounce. My grandmother-in-law told me to start him on formula, so we did and never looked back. My baby finally started sleeping.

I Bounced Back Really Fast

I was miserable and sore for several days. I had cleavage for the first time in my life when my milk came in. I hurt, but I had great boobs! I had a great six week maternity leave and bounced back really fast. For a first time mom, I did well except I was up-tight about pumping at work and I was sore. I had a friend who belonged to a Le Leche group and she talked me through a few struggles. Finally, my daughter weaned herself at seven months. I think she was unfulfilled, so I supplemented with formula. She was allergic to everything but Alimentum. My biggest surprise was that I was more ready for motherhood than I'd ever thought I could be. I was 30 when my first child was born. I raised her while I held a full time job. We traveled with Dad on the weekends for his job. She has come into her own as a world traveler/adventure seeker with her husband.

Breastfeeding Was Hard

I was very emotional. I felt like I cried a lot, but it passed. I had a lot of support from our family and husband. Breastfeeding lasted about four months with my first pregnancy. It only lasted three months with my daughter because she had horrible stomach issues and I literally couldn't eat anything that didn't upset her. We finally had to switch her to Alimentum formula and she was an entirely different baby. Finally, with my twins, I literally tried my hardest. Since I knew it was my last pregnancy, I was all in.

Breastfeeding twins was so hard. One twin would only take my breast, the other one wouldn't take it at all and I had to pump and feed. We literally tried everything to get him to latch. He Just wouldn't. I said it was just because he was lazy. The constant pumping and worry about having enough for him and for the other twin just got to be too much. I wasn't producing as much, so I just stopped after three months.

Postpartum Was Horrible

I was pregnant and gave birth in 2008 and there was a complete lack of support for mothers in the community and workplace. I felt no emotion whatsoever when I first saw my baby. I had severe postpartum depression due to a traumatic birth. I didn't get a chance to breastfeed, as I was not given proper education. The nurses said they already started him on bottle feeding due to my emergency C-section and my being sedated, and they said it was "too late" to breastfeed. Postpartum was horrible. I had no support and ended up giving temporary custody to my mother. I spiraled into an alcoholic depression.

One Day at a Time

Honestly, dealing with recovery from having a C-section and partial hysterectomy, and my three beautiful babies being in the NICU for two months, I didn't have time to think about the postpartum. I just got through each day the best I could. I actually got "shamed" by a lot of people -- mostly nurses because I didn't plan on breastfeeding. It was a choice my husband and I made when we found out about having triplets. Nobody talked to me about freezing my milk and putting it into bottles. I probably would have then. We just knew we didn't want it just being me having to feed all three babies, especially since I had a full time job. I knew I would love those babies with all my heart, but didn't know it would fill my heart so much that I couldn't even breathe the first time I held them.

Part Two

My Story

The following chapters are my story and the inspiration for this book. I started writing as a way to help process my own experiences and put into words what I was feeling. One thing I realized is that I will always be processing it in one way or another. Your feelings about your birth experiences can change over time, even day by day. It never ceases to amaze me that we can feel so many things at once. Some days I feel proud and empowered; other days I feel guilty and I'm left questioning myself.

I always knew I would love my children deeply. But I never imagined how birth could be so much more than bringing your child into the world. You not only give birth to your child, you give birth to a new version of yourself.

My Daughter's Birth

When it comes to a big life event like becoming a parent, so many feelings can coexist. I distinctly remember feeling so happy to meet my baby. But I also felt apprehensive about the whole experience. There were so many aspects about childbirth that were out of my control, and I didn't like that I couldn't predict what would happen.

I was a very anxious first time mom. During my whole pregnancy I was just nervous about everything, way more than I should have been. I had an unhealthy obsession with trying to learn as much as I could about the process to prepare for every single scenario. Thinking and planning about how this baby was going to come out of me was such a daunting task.

When I was about 37 weeks along, I started having some discomfort while I was at work. I thought, "Is this the beginning of labor? This might be happening!" I felt a lot of tightness, and it got to the point where I was so uncomfortable that I couldn't even sit at my desk anymore. I wound up standing while taking calls for most of the day. Towards the end of the work day, I was getting anxious about this possibly being labor.

I started walking up the steps to tell my husband, when I felt a big movement. To this day I still have a hard time describing this sensation. I looked down, and my belly just looked like a wave while I felt a big "plop." I noticed that the tight feeling had gone away, and I just assumed it was all a false alarm.

My 38 week appointment was a couple days later. My doctor had a puzzled look on his face as he felt my belly. He said, "It feels like your baby's butt is in your pelvis today. We're going to bring in the portable ultrasound and check her positioning."

My heart dropped. I started to think about our very first prenatal appointment when I asked my doctor what would happen if our baby was breech. Back then he said, "Oh, it's way too early to worry about that." But I think I knew even then; I just had a gut feeling.

I also thought about how active our baby was throughout my whole pregnancy. We had to get three separate ultrasounds just to find out her gender and get all the pictures the doctors needed to be sure she was healthy. She was never in the same position during any of them. I remember during one ultrasound the technician took the wand off for one moment, and when she put it back she said, "What in the world? Did your baby just flip around? She did!" She told us that we had the most active fetus she had ever seen.

Our doctor brought in the portable ultrasound, and sure enough, she was breech. I just sat there dumbfounded. My doctor asked, "Are you okay?" and I just burst into tears. I was completely devastated because I knew what this would mean. I was really hoping and preparing for a natural birth, and it looked like that plan had gone out the window. I was absolutely terrified of having surgery. I asked if there was any way we could try to turn our baby, and he offered to try an external cephalic version (ECV) in the next few days, but if that didn't work, he would recommend a cesarean.

We still made a plan for a vaginal birth, but we also made one for a cesarean. My doctor made sure to answer all of our questions and concerns. I researched everything I could about cesareans to try to prepare myself the days leading up to the ECV. I told my doctor that all I really wanted was for my arms to be free so that I could hold my daughter right away if it was possible. He said he couldn't promise my arms wouldn't be strapped down because it was the anesthesiologist's choice, but he would do his best to ask. That's when I told him, "If my arms are strapped to the table and I don't get to hold my baby right away, I'm going to throw a fit." I was pretty adamant about that, and it didn't help that my pregnancy hormones were totally out of whack at that point.

Two days before my ECV I had some bleeding and more cramping, so I decided to go to the hospital to be monitored. After about a half an hour of being there, the nurse came back into the room somewhat panicked and said, "You didn't tell me your baby is breech!" I didn't think it was a big deal, but her reaction made me feel otherwise. She asked me if I was feeling any of the contractions I was having and I told her I wasn't. She said that they were going to keep me for a couple hours to see if the contractions got closer together. She seemed nervous, which made me nervous. Was my baby in danger?

We were there for two hours before they finally decided to let us go home. As she discharged us, she told me to avoid anything that could bring on labor. "You don't want to go into labor with a breech baby." I didn't understand what the big deal was, other than they probably wouldn't try the ECV if I was in labor. Why couldn't I go into labor if the only problem was that my baby was facing the wrong way? I was determined to have them try to flip her around.

I remember one of my mom's friends told me, "Breech is just a variation of normal." I kept hearing that phrase, but I didn't understand what it meant. If breech is so normal, then why doesn't anyone act like it is? I tried everything I could to naturally turn our baby back around. I tried swimming, chiropractic care, Spinning Babies exercises, ice packs, playing music low on my belly, and even standing on my head. I tried talking to my baby and asking her to turn head down. Needless to say, none of that worked, and I knew we were going to try the ECV.

I remember sleeping fine the night before the ECV. I felt like I was making the right decision and I was doing everything in my power to get my baby here safely. The next day, as we drove to the hospital, I still felt calm. It was when I walked through the hospital doors that I suddenly didn't feel okay anymore. Everything started to feel more real. I felt this deep sense of dread. This wasn't what I wanted. I tried to ignore it as we continued down the hall and into the room.

I had to do what was best for my baby. There was an illusion of control, of options. We would try turning my baby with the ECV. The fact that I had no other options other than a C-section if the ECV didn't work was a trauma all in itself. I brought my whole family to the hospital with us, which in hindsight was probably a terrible idea. I just felt like we needed all the support we could get.

The ECV was supposed to be at 9:00 that morning. But it got moved to 11:00 a.m., which turned to 1:00 p.m. I was not happy about it being pushed back so many times. I was so incredibly thirsty and hungry because they wouldn't let me eat or drink anything. My husband kept sneaking me sips of water every chance he could. I was just so uncomfortable and felt dizzy.

The nurse tried putting an IV in my arm, and I asked her to place it in my hand instead. She ignored my request and continued trying to put it in my forearm, which blew a vein. A combination of that, my fear of needles, and low blood sugar caused me to faint. She apologized to me, but I just stared off into space. I felt like I was trapped. I wanted to go back home or be anywhere else.

Another nurse came in and told me it was time to place a bladder catheter. I just stared at her while she opened the package and tried to get it ready, all while my entire family was in the room. This was something that came as a total surprise. I asked, "Right now? Can't this wait until after I get an epidural or something?" She told me, "It has to be now. I'm sorry."

As someone who experienced a sexual assault, the thought of having this done without any medication paralyzed me.

I felt like none of my requests and feelings mattered. I was too afraid to speak up again, and I was visibly upset. My husband insisted that the catheter be placed later. The nurse went to ask the doctor, and thankfully he said it was all right to wait. I felt out of control, like a passenger in a car. Things were just being done to me instead of my doing something important to bring my child into the world. I felt like I was on autopilot, and when they asked if I was okay with having students in the room, I said yes. As time went on, I became more and more anxious.

When the nurse came in to see how I was doing, I started crying. She gave me a big hug and told me I was doing great and everything would be okay. I was wheeled into the OR, and I was so scared that I thought about running away. The room was a lot bigger than I expected, and they were playing pop music, which I thought was odd. I didn't even notice that my husband was no longer with me when I got on the table. My doctor asked me where my husband was and I didn't know. It turns out they had him wait in another room so they could get me prepared for the procedure.

I was not prepared to be in a room full of people I didn't know while they placed the epidural. It was traumatic. There were nurses, doctors, and students, but my husband wasn't allowed. It seemed so unfair. This was just another day for these people, but it was all new and scary to me. I cried the whole time.

My anesthesiologist was nice and tried to keep me calm. However, I couldn't help being upset. I was upset about being talked down to like a child, and that I was going through this scary procedure alone. They had a difficult time inserting the epidural. If I could have just had my husband with me, it would have helped keep me calm. It took them around 40 minutes to get my epidural in, and I blame it on not being able to relax. Everything went by in a blur. At one point the upper part of my body went numb, and I fainted from sudden low blood pressure. It was the worst sensation in the world.

During this time, my husband walked up to the OR window and all he could see was my hand hanging off the side of the bed. He panicked and asked another nurse what was going on. He thought I was dead. They finally decided to let my husband in the room. To this day, that memory still upsets him. He experienced trauma from this event too.

Once the ultrasound was set up, they checked my baby's position and fluid levels. Everything was ready for the ECV. I couldn't catch my breath as the two doctors started pushing on my belly to try and turn my baby. They tried to turn her for about 10 minutes, but it felt like an eternity. I watched as beads of sweat started forming on their brows. They seemed to be using all of their strength as they pushed. It wasn't painful, but it was very intense.

Suddenly, our baby's heart rate dropped. The doctors immediately took their hands off of my belly, and everyone held their breath and watched the monitor. Relief came over all of us when her heart rate bounced back. That was when my doctor told me, "I'm really sorry, but I think a cesarean would be our best option from here." I was so exhausted from all the pushing on my belly and the hectic day. I agreed, and I felt that it was the right choice.

The curtain went up and I felt a lot of pulling and tugging, so much that I felt like I was about to fall off the table. I was thankful I didn't have my arms in restraints, as I found myself grabbing onto the sides of the table for dear life. At that point, I began to understand why they typically strap your arms down. My doctor asked me through the drape how I was doing, and I told him, "I feel like I'm being scooped out like a pumpkin!" Everyone had a chuckle at that.

The anesthesiologist asked my husband if he wanted to look over the curtain and watch our daughter be born. He did for about a minute, and I thought that was so brave! I expected to hear silence on the other side of the curtain because I was always told babies born by cesarean don't cry right away. When my daughter was pulled out, she cried immediately. They briefly showed her to me over the curtain and whisked her away to the warmer. I could barely see her, though, as everything was blurry because I wasn't allowed to wear my glasses.

She cried and cried and I wanted to go to her. I waited anxiously while I heard her screaming behind the curtain. It felt like I was sort of disconnected from it all. Did I really just give birth? It didn't feel like it. The anesthesiologist brought a TV screen next to the head of the table so I could see the nurses clean her off. This helped me feel less disoriented since I could finally see what was going on.

I was completely shocked to see her legs were still stuck all the way up by her head, with her feet bent towards her shins. At first I couldn't even see her feet at all, and I worried that she might not have any. Then the nurse straightened them out, and I was so relieved to see that she did, in fact, have feet.

I couldn't wait to finally hold and meet this little person who had been growing in my belly the past nine months. I was starting to feel a little distressed by how much our daughter was crying and told my husband to go to her. She cried the whole time until she was finally placed on my chest. She immediately looked into my eyes and stopped crying. I could tell she knew who I was, and it was such an amazing feeling. We just stared at each other while I held her. She looked so beautiful and wise. I just couldn't believe she was mine.

It wasn't long before I started shaking and I felt like I couldn't hold our daughter anymore. I passed her off to my husband and the anesthesiologist told him he would give me something to "relax" me through my IV. I immediately lost consciousness, which shocked my husband, and he asked if I was okay. The anesthesiologist assured him that I was fine and that he could take our daughter back to the room. I was not expecting them to give me medications like this without asking me first. It felt like another thing I had no control over.

I was sort of in and out of consciousness as they wheeled me into the recovery room. I stared at the ceiling, and all I could feel was my shaking. I couldn't move my arms or any part of my body, but at the same time I felt myself shaking uncontrollably. I didn't know if it was because of the medications, or if I was in shock from the day's experiences. Everything was out of my control. When one of the nurses tried to reassure me that my shaking was normal, I tried to open my mouth to speak, but couldn't. It was such a scary feeling. At this point, I was determined that I would never go through this again.

When I was taken back to my room, I tried to get up and walk right away. The nurses came in and caught me as I almost fell out of bed. They couldn't believe I could feel my legs already. I felt desperate to get up and move. I just needed to get out of that bed. I couldn't stand the inflating boots they had put on my legs, or the bladder catheter any more. The anxiety of not being in control of anything was getting to me, and I panicked. When my family took pictures of us holding our daughter, I could barely smile.

A few hours later I was given the okay to walk the halls with my husband. We stopped at a collage of beautiful birth announcements that was hanging on the wall, and I started to cry. I always imagined walking those halls while I was in labor, having my husband help me breathe through each contraction. I felt like the choice to deliver my baby naturally had been taken from me. I didn't think I would feel so sad about it once my daughter was here.

I never thought that I could feel happy she was here and healthy and still be shocked and sad that things hadn't gone the way I had hoped. Even with all the preparation for this birth, I still felt traumatized by some of it. I felt robbed. It was such a conflicting feeling. Despite my feelings, I knew this was the right birth for her, and it was still beautiful and perfect in its own way.

Becoming a Doula

After having my first child, I was surprised by how little support I felt over my feelings. People told me, "At least you have a healthy baby," but I didn't feel healthy myself. I was hurting emotionally and physically. I mourned over the birth I had hoped for and grieved over not even getting a chance to go into labor. I truly felt "less than" because of it. I felt that I wasn't a good mother because I was sad about how my daughter came into the world.

A few weeks after the birth, I was speaking to a doula about my experience and she said matter of factly, "A breech baby isn't a reason for a C-section, you know. You just didn't try hard enough to avoid it." She was someone who was supposed to provide unbiased support, but her words cut me to my core.

So many other people said, "At least you can schedule the next one," or, "At least you don't have to experience labor." At least, at least, at least. It drove me crazy. Whenever I expressed my feelings of grief over my experience, there was always someone who came back with, "Other people have it worse," or, "At least you can get pregnant, just be grateful."

Even though I would consider my daughter's birth a positive one, I still had some trauma from it. Now that I've had plenty of time to reflect on this, I understand that no one wanted to hurt me that day. The lack of control I felt, and the sense that things were just being done to my body, triggered feelings from a past assault. I can acknowledge that this was not anyone's intention, while also acknowledging my own feelings towards it. At the time, I didn't feel that I even gave birth. Part of me struggled to believe this baby was mine. I loved her dearly, but I felt disconnected from her and the whole experience.

Postpartum depression was really bad. I had anxiety before she was born, but it became worse afterwards. One evening, while waiting for my husband to come back from work, I put a casserole in the oven. Out of sheer exhaustion and panic, I thought I had placed my baby in there instead. I felt like I had no sense of reality, and I didn't trust myself to be alone with my baby. I called my mom, and she asked me to make my daughter cry so she could hear her and make sure she was okay. That experience terrified me and made me question having more kids in the future.

One night I told my husband that I didn't want any other children because I was so afraid of having another C-section. Our daughter would be an only child. I will never forget the look in his eyes when he asked me if I was sure. We always talked about having at least two or three children. Saying that I couldn't see myself having another C-section broke his heart. The truth was, I wasn't sure. A part of me had thought about having a VBAC, even while I had been on the operating table. I was just afraid.

A few weeks after this painful conversation with my husband, I saw an advertisement for International Cesarean Awareness Network (ICAN). They were having a meeting in the city, and I just knew I had to go. My husband was such a good sport because he came with me. All the women told their cesarean and VBAC stories, and it was eye opening. One woman had a vaginal birth after three cesareans, which I never even knew was possible. When it was my turn to tell my story, I broke down in tears. Everyone was supportive and validated how I felt. Talking to the group gave me hope and inspired me. I don't believe I would have pursued doula work if I didn't meet these women.

I felt that I was armed with knowledge because I knew my options for my future births. To my surprise whenever I brought up VBAC to anyone local to me, no one seemed to know what it was, including some of the medical professionals I knew. I found it very problematic that mothers who had a primary cesarean were then told that their future births needed to be cesareans. They were also told they could only have three cesareans total. It was as if the medical system was dictating how many children these parents were "allowed" to have, and it didn't sit right with me. Some hospitals had "VBAC bans," which shocked me. How can you ban birth? I told everyone I knew that VBAC was possible and a safe option.

I became very vocal about VBAC on social media, and at first I got a lot of backlash. People told me it didn't matter how your baby is born and didn't understand why I wouldn't just go along with what doctors said. It was apparent to me that VBAC access was a women's rights issue. Hospitals having VBAC bans means mandated surgery on mothers with a prior cesarean. How can anyone give consent to a repeat cesarean if they can't say no? There was a fire in me.

I called my local hospital and wrote a letter asking them to reconsider their policies. I pestered my doctor at every visit asking if the hospital was allowing VBAC. Other mothers sent me messages or called me asking about VBAC. I told them to talk to their doctors about it and referred them to hospitals that allowed it. I did this for almost four years, until I finally heard that my local hospital lifted their ban. I'm not sure that I can take the credit, but I would like to think I played a role in it.

There are so many options for birth that are not always presented to mothers. Learning about VBAC and the different choices we have fueled my passion to become a doula. The start of my doula training was with an agency of several other doulas. The first birth I ever attended was for a first time mom who had a fast, unmedicated labor. I was able to shadow another doula and I was just trying to stay out of everyone's way. This mother had her baby within five minutes of us showing up! It was amazing to see how normal childbirth could be.

The second birth I attended reconfirmed that doula work was what I was called to do. I was called in as a backup at the last minute, so I didn't know much about the mother other than her name. As I was introducing myself to the mother, a nurse came in to ask her a few questions. The nurse asked, "I have here that you had two cesareans, is that right?" The mother said, "Yes, I'm going for a VBAC." I froze, waiting for someone to recommend a repeat C-section, but it didn't happen. The hospital staff treated it like any other birth. It was empowering to be a part of her birth story as she had a successful vaginal birth after two cesareans.

Every birth I went to seemed to heal the part of me that desired to experience it all myself. I found my calling. However, a little part of me still felt like a fraud. During one of the childbirth classes I was teaching, a mother asked, "What does a contraction feel like?" I didn't know what to say at first as I couldn't give her an honest answer. Who would want a doula who had never even felt a contraction? I truly felt that I missed a rite of passage by not even experiencing labor. I really had a lot of emotional baggage to sort through.

My daughter's birth stirred up a lot of negative feelings about myself. I felt that my body was defective, that I did not really give birth to my daughter and that I could not protect her. I was constantly worried that she was going to get hurt or die. I felt like an awful mother. I sought out therapy to work through what I was feeling.

Along with the emotional trauma, I had unexplained physical pain that lasted for three years after my daughter's birth. It felt like a rubber band was constricting on the right side of my abdomen down to my right hip. There was also nerve pain that felt like an electric shock whenever the weather would change. It was so bad that I saw several different doctors for it. At one point, the pain was so intense that I found myself in the emergency room. The doctor initially thought that I had appendicitis, but after running tests they couldn't find an explanation for my pain.

I finally decided to see a pelvic pain specialist, who introduced me to the idea that my pain could be caused from the scar tissue due to my C-section. She told me it was possible that scar tissue fused to my bladder or bowel. I had no idea that could happen or that this was one of the risks of having surgery. Prior to this visit, there was hardly any information given to me on how to heal from a cesarean. It was disappointing that it took so long to figure out what was potentially wrong with me.

The specialist sent me to physical therapy, and it changed my outlook on everything. Working on my physical healing after my cesarean had such an impact on me. My treatment plan included releasing the scar tissue. I was always jumpy whenever anyone would get near that part of my body. It felt like a cruel joke to wind up with a scar there. For me, healing emotionally was just as important as healing physically.

After weeks of exercises to help work through the scar tissue, I left my last appointment in tears. I wasn't in pain anymore, and for the first time in my life, I thought that I really could add to our family. I realized my journey over the past few years, from learning about VBAC and working as a doula, to the physical therapy, had provided healing for me. I suddenly realized it would be okay, no matter how the next birth played out.

My Son's Birth

I started off my second pregnancy believing everything was going to work out perfectly. I had my heart set on a VBAC, and our local rural hospital had recently lifted their ban. It had been almost five years since I had my first baby, and I just knew my body and this baby were going to be different. I was determined to make this VBAC work, so I started chiropractic care and Spinning Babies exercises right away. I was constantly trying to feel my baby's position using Belly Mapping, and I knew something didn't feel right, but since I always felt his hiccups down low in my pelvis, I had a false sense of security.

It was a little bit of a shock during my 34 week ultrasound when we found that this baby was also breech. He also still had a nuchal cord that was present since the 20 week scan. The ultrasound technician said, "It doesn't look like your little guy wants to come out," which annoyed me. I knew breech babies could be born vaginally; the trick was finding someone experienced and willing to do it.

My prenatal appointment was right after the ultrasound, and I told my doctor what happened before he even had the chance to look at the results. I asked him if there was any way we could deliver this baby naturally. He told me he had some training with it but explained the risks and that the hospital's malpractice insurance doesn't allow it. I couldn't believe I was in this situation again. It was standard to schedule a C-section at around 39 to 40 weeks, but I didn't feel right about doing that. I knew that I was not going to willingly schedule another C-section just because my baby was facing the wrong way. If there were some other health issues, that would have been another story. However, my baby was not in imminent danger just because he wanted to come out butt first.

As my doctor was going over my options, I blurted out, "Well, what if I refuse?" He asked if I meant, "Refuse the C-section?" I felt myself get quiet as I realized how absurd I sounded. He seemed to be taken aback by this but said, "I wouldn't be mad." He explained that they would probably try to send me to another hospital if I was stable enough and refused a C-section.

Breech babies can be born vaginally, this much I knew. There are a lot of success stories out there, but there are also a lot of horror stories.

At this point I didn't actually want to refuse the C-section, I just did not feel right about scheduling my baby's birthday. I wanted to give him time to turn head down and be ready to come out. I wanted to labor. The thought of scheduling a C-section again made my skin crawl, thinking about the anxiety leading up to that day and how I would have to go hours without any water and feeling sick and out of control again. I was afraid my preferences with this birth wouldn't be respected. I couldn't do it. I wouldn't schedule it. And this time I knew no one could make me. There was a lot of unresolved trauma coming to the surface.

We decided to try the ECV again and my doctor wasted no time scheduling one in the city with a doctor who had a high success rate. My doctor called me with the details of the ECV and told me that the baby was complete breech, which made the chances of success a little higher. Then he reiterated that if it didn't work, he would recommend a C-section.

That's when I asked him point blank if he had ever even seen a vaginal breech delivery. He told me he had, but it had been a long time. This confirmed that going to the hospital in labor and refusing a C-section would not be a wise thing to do. If this ECV didn't work, I would have to resign myself to the fact that I would just have to have a cesarean.

Despite all of that, I was feeling really good about the ECV. I was also still trying everything I could to flip this baby around myself. At the consult for the ECV, the doctor checked my fluid levels and my baby's position. He said everything looked good except that my baby was now in Frank breech position, which is not ideal but still possible to turn with the ECV.

My first baby was also Frank breech, and her ECV had failed, so hearing that was slightly annoying. Despite that news, I still had high hopes that this could work. The ECV was scheduled two days after the consultation. My husband and I stayed in a hotel the night before so that we wouldn't have to get up at 4:00 a.m. and drive an hour away. I got up early and started working on forward leaning inversions on the couch as a last ditch effort to help my baby move during the procedure.

When we got to the hospital they started the consent forms right away, and before I knew it, the anesthesiologist was in. I decided to get an epidural because it would increase the chances that my baby would turn. My husband got to be with me when they placed it, which was different from my daughter's birth.

From here, things got a little crazy. My blood pressure immediately plummeted, and the nurse had to call someone in to give me something to stabilize it. My blood pressure continued to drop several times throughout the procedure. They kept giving me more and more medication to help bring it back up. I also had to wear a mask the whole time because this was during the pandemic. It made it even worse when I already felt so short of breath.

The doctor came in to do another ultrasound before starting and said that my fluid levels dropped from 10 to 6. He seemed very concerned with such a sharp drop in just two days. He asked if my water broke or if I was leaking fluid. I told him that I didn't notice anything like that.

As he was talking to me, he had another doctor check my cervix to see if I was dilated. I wasn't even aware that this was happening because I was numb from the epidural and couldn't move. I did not appreciate the lack of communication and the sense that they could do whatever they wanted with my body without asking.

Once they determined that I wasn't dilated or leaking fluid at all, the doctor told me that this procedure probably wasn't going to work now, but he could still try anyway. I asked him to try since I already went through the trouble of getting an epidural.

In between my blood pressure dropping, the two doctors tried to turn my baby. One of them told me if I needed them to stop, just to say so and they would stop immediately. It was an intense pressure but not painful. I never told them to stop because I wanted it to work so badly. They tried twice, and on the second time, they almost got my baby's head into my pelvis. Once his little head passed my hip bone, it was as if they hit some kind of resistance, and he bounced back to being breech.

The doctor told me he was sorry and that he recommended another ultrasound in a week. He explained that if my fluid levels were 5 or below, it was time to deliver. I didn't say a word and just rolled over in the hospital bed. I was exhausted and my blood pressure still wouldn't cooperate. At that moment, I felt so defeated and broken.

I cried the rest of the day because this was my last chance. With all the drama of my blood pressure dropping during the epidural, I was terrified of going through all of that again. It reconfirmed the fact that I couldn't schedule a C-section. The fear of it all made me determined to find a provider to help me deliver this baby naturally.

For the next two weeks, I was sick with anxiety. I frequently woke up in the middle of the night with panic attacks about a surgery I did not want. I did not feel safe giving birth anywhere. I hated that even though we were in good health, I had this C-section looming over my head. I felt traumatized by not having any other choices.

I continued to try things to turn him naturally. I did moxibustion, acupuncture, music low on my belly, ice high on my belly, essential oils, a homeopathic remedy called pulsatilla and hypnosis. The list of things I tried was a mile long. I tried talking to my son just like I did with my daughter, begging him to just turn head down, but I wound up feeling stupid.

I reached out to two different homebirth midwives to see if they would help me. One of them had several years of experience, but she lived three hours away, and the other one said she needed another midwife's assistance if I were to hire her for a breech birth. It was getting pretty late in the pregnancy, and I was running out of time to find someone.

I had one of the midwives do a prenatal visit with me. She listened to my baby's heart using a pinard stethoscope and checked my blood pressure. She checked my baby's positioning while I laid on the couch, and she frowned. She said, "Your baby is transverse today, not breech." Great. My baby seemed to be getting into a worse position every day. It explained all the discomfort I had been feeling the past couple days.

She offered to try some techniques in an attempt to give my baby more space to move head down. She had me get on my hands and knees and used the rebozo to "sift" my belly. Then she told me to crawl around on the floor and had me lean forward on hands and knees while she used the rebozo to sift around my sacrum. We did this several times for about an hour.

I felt ridiculous, but did it anyway because I was desperate for something to work. My husband just scratched his head as he watched us. The last time I crawled along the floor, I felt a big movement. I let the midwife know, so she checked my baby's position again and she said, "Well, he's breech but he's actually in a better position than before." I was skeptical, but I did feel better afterwards. We thanked the midwife as she left. My husband looked at me and asked, "You're not seriously thinking about having a home birth, are you?" Truth be told, I wasn't sure. I felt a lot safer in a hospital setting, especially if my baby was breech.

I called the other midwife who lived three hours away to get a better idea of how a homebirth would look. I asked if there was anything else I could try to turn my baby. She said, "If you've tried everything in your power, the next best exercise is acceptance. Your baby is probably breech for a reason." I was on the fence about it all, but, ultimately, I didn't feel right about having a home birth.

I cried every day thinking about how I would be expected to schedule a C-section. I knew in my heart that I could not schedule my baby's birthday. I wasn't able to make an appointment with my doctor during this time. My anxiety was high and I was physically and emotionally exhausted. Then, of course, there was the stress of the pandemic on top of all of this. I wasn't sure what to do. I just wanted to feel safe.

I was in so much denial about a C-section happening, that I decided to call every hospital in the city to see if anyone would take a VBAC breech. I was told "no" probably a hundred times. So I was surprised to get a call back from a doctor who was willing to discuss it with me. Without hesitation, I scheduled a meeting with her. I wasn't expecting her to take me on as a patient so late in my pregnancy, but I was somewhat hopeful and curious about what she had to say. Ironically, I never got to meet with this doctor, as my son decided to be born before we could have our scheduled meeting.

Two days later, I woke up feeling a little off and I couldn't put my finger on why. I just felt different. I had finally been able to schedule the ultrasound to check my fluid levels, and I was nervous about the results. Would I get a call back saying I needed a C-section this week? What if my fluid levels were too low and our baby really was in danger? I was so emotional about it.

I had been having mild contractions for a couple of days but brushed them off. As my husband and I were on our way to the appointment, I had a big contraction and dropped my cell phone on the concrete, shattering the screen. It was unusable. I was so upset because it was a brand new phone and I was afraid that the hospital wouldn't be able to get a hold of me if the ultrasound results were bad.

When we got to the hospital at 8:00 a.m. I started noticing contractions even more. It was two weeks until my due date, so I kept telling myself it was nothing to worry about. I used my husband's cell phone to make a zoom call with my therapist in the hospital parking lot. I unloaded a lot of my fears about the ultrasound and the upcoming birth in general. I started feeling the contractions more, but I attributed them to my being so upset.

When I went in for my ultrasound an hour later, I had to breathe through a couple of the contractions. It was very obvious to the ultrasound tech, and she asked if I was alright. I told her that I was just having some Braxton Hicks contractions but I was fine.

143

She quickly took the pictures and sent us on our way saying, "Maybe next time you're here, you'll have the baby!" I didn't realize that would be true at the time. I also went into the chiropractor for a last minute adjustment while we were in town. They could also tell I was in early labor, even though I was in denial. They excitedly squeezed me into their schedule and wished me luck.

Then my husband and I quickly ran to Verizon to see if they could do anything about my phone, but all they could do at the time was put an insurance claim on it. I dealt with not having a working phone all day and it annoyed me.

As I sat in my home office, trying to work, I got more and more annoyed. I was just irritated by everything. I did a few interviews with my work phone and had to pause a couple of times during one of them just to breathe. That's when I realized I should probably be timing the contractions.

By the time 5 o'clock rolled around, I couldn't focus. I ran down stairs and told my husband that we needed to go to Verizon again and switch out my phone to another one that worked. He didn't seem to feel the urgency that I did, but with all these contractions, I knew something was up. We got to Verizon and I was contracting more. At this point, I had been timing them at 7 minutes apart on the dot. Luckily, I was able to switch out my phone quickly and we picked up dinner.

I had never experienced real contractions with my first, so I wasn't 100% sure what to expect. I decided to call my doula to tell her what was going on. As we were driving home, she said it would be a good idea to call the hospital and consider going in once my contractions picked up to 5-7 minutes apart since this baby was breech and they would need time to set up the OR.

I got silent for a moment. Mine were already 7 minutes apart and getting closer together, but we were headed home, the opposite direction of the hospital. I told my husband, "I think we need to turn around." He asked, "Are you serious?" I said, "Well, I don't know."

I didn't know what to do. I certainly didn't want to put our baby at risk by staying home too long. We didn't end up hiring that midwife, and at this rate, I wasn't sure if she would even make it to our home in time. Our doula reassured us not to panic and suggested I take a bath when we got home to see if it would slow things down.

We picked up our daughter from my parents' house and then I immediately hopped in the tub. I called my mom to tell her what was going on, and during that 10 minute call, I barely spoke because I had three contractions. The tub was picking things up, not slowing them down. I hung up with her and quickly ran down stairs because I knew we were going to the hospital.

I wanted to eat dinner before we went because there was no way I was going to be starving myself before having this baby. Who knows if this was even the real thing anyway? I scarfed down my food, and after my last bite, I felt that my contractions were getting significantly stronger and closer together. My poor daughter ran up to me and asked, "Mommy, play with me?" over and over, but I couldn't focus. Things turned into a blur of chaos.

All of a sudden, I yelled at my husband to pack the bags and get things going. He asked how far apart my contractions were, and I wasn't keeping count at that point. After he worked on the bags for a bit, my husband looked at me in terror and said, "Babe, they're 3 minutes apart right now." I panicked and started frantically cleaning the bathroom. My husband asked what on Earth I was doing, and I told him, "I have to clean this place!"

My doula was on the phone again and she said, "Don't worry about your bags, you need to get out the door now!" I continued frantically cleaning as I was having contractions, and my husband had to basically carry me out the door.

I called my mom and told her we were once again dropping our daughter off and heading to the hospital. My husband drove 75 m.p.h. all the way there as my doula was on speaker phone coaching me through contractions. We almost hit a skunk on the road, and I screamed at my husband to swerve and miss it. Then we hit a pheasant. The drive alone was an adventure!

We finally made it to the hospital and I stepped out of the van. My doula told me to just take a moment, so I stood with my hands on the side of the van. I didn't want to go in because I knew it would mean another C-section if this boy didn't miraculously flip around. As much as I was convinced that I would make it closer to 40 weeks, I could no longer deny that this was the real thing.

We walked inside. The receptionist and a very nice nurse met us at the entrance. Before they could say anything, I told them, "Hi, I'm in labor!" They both offered me a wheelchair and I yelled, "No, I don't need it!" I was having excruciating back labor and I couldn't stand putting any pressure on it.

As we walked to the elevator, I burst into tears and asked the nurse, "Is my doctor going to be here?" She said that he was on call for me and she

145

would let him know I was there. I was scared, so it was a relief to have someone there I knew and trusted.

On the way up to the L&D floor I said, "You know, maybe this isn't the real thing. Maybe it's just indigestion and I can go home." The nurse said, "Honey, I don't think so. I'm pretty sure you're in labor." I was hooked up to the monitors, and my contractions were around 3 to 4 minutes apart. The nurse tried to check me but couldn't reach my cervix, so she called another nurse to help. After what felt like several minutes of her checking, the nurse determined I was around 2 cm dilated.

They kept me for observation as I continued cursing through contractions for a few more hours. I was surprised to feel my contractions were mostly concentrated in my lower back and along my previous cesarean scar.

After a few hours, the nurse told me she called my doctor and he thought I might be having "uterine irritability" and that they might send me home if the IV fluids helped calm things down. At this point, I almost lost it. I could not believe that I was being dramatic over fake contractions! I was so sure that this was real labor, and I could not imagine being sent home like this. The nurse decided to switch up the monitors, and it showed that my contractions were 2 to 3 minutes apart.

The nurses tried to check me again, but neither of them could reach my cervix to tell how far along I was. I took that as a sign that I wasn't progressing through all of this. Truth be told, I didn't really want to make any progress just because I knew it would mean that I would be going in for a C-section. However, it would have been nice to know that these awful contractions were doing something productive.

The contractions felt like they were right on top of each other, and I was going mad. No matter what position I tried, hands and knees, kneeling, on the birth ball, or in the shower, nothing helped to ease the pain. It was exhausting. I tried to sleep through the contractions, but I would get so uncomfortable that I wanted to scream. My husband and the nurse reminded me to breathe through them, but it was so hard.

A few weeks prior, my doula had given my husband a list of things to do for comfort techniques because she couldn't be there. During labor, I was surprised to find that I didn't want any of them. I was even more surprised to find myself screaming at my husband to get away from me. I didn't want to be touched at all because I found it to be so painful. I always imagined my husband would be by my side the whole time during labor, but I felt

146

better being completely alone. Sometimes I still get disappointed when I think about this. I never meant to exclude him from the process.

There came a point where I was just sick of the contractions and screamed into the quiet room, "Go away!" I got up to use the bathroom and had a big contraction. My scar felt like it was about to tear open, and a lot of pressure was released. I felt a gush and I was sure my uterus ruptured. I was afraid to look down. I was afraid I would either see blood or meconium. I was relieved to see that it was clear. It was just my water breaking. Ironically, I didn't have any contractions for several minutes after this, but it wasn't long before they would pick up again.

I went to the bathroom and looked at myself in the mirror. I looked like a disheveled mess. I wasn't keeping track of time at that point, but I would later realize that my entire labor was over 24 hours. It felt as if I was going to keep having contractions until I died. I reluctantly called the nurse, and she told me she would call the doctor right away. I knew what was coming next.

Shortly after, my doctor came into the room while I was on the floor having another contraction. He sat in a chair next to me and told me that I did a good job with labor so far, but for safety reasons, from the baby being breech and my water breaking, he recommended a cesarean.

My mind skipped from each scenario. If I refused, they could send us somewhere else. Where would that even be? I knew for a fact that no hospital in a 90 mile radius would take a breech VBAC because I had called every one of them. If something bad happened, my baby would probably be sent to a NICU an hour away. Things could go wrong really quickly. I could either consent to the C-section, or wait until it was a real emergency.

My top priority was to get my baby here safely. I really wanted to wait until he was ready to be born, and I had gotten to do that. I wanted my choices to be respected, and they were. No one was going to force me to do anything I didn't want to do. I wanted to avoid a traumatic birth, but most of all I wanted to avoid a tragic outcome. After all, I got pregnant to have a baby, not just a birth experience.

My doctor continued to acknowledge how he knew this wasn't what I wanted and he was sorry. I think he wanted me to have this VBAC just as much as I did. After having another contraction and finding out that after 10 hours of laboring in the hospital, I was still only at 2 cm, I cried, "Why is my body doing the opposite of what it's supposed to do? Why is it failing me?"

My doctor reassured me that my body was doing exactly what it was supposed to and that I was in the natural process of labor, my baby was just in the wrong position. I had another contraction as he apologized again. I told him, "It's fine, I'm about ready to cut him out myself!" I never thought I would say something like this in a million years, and I think it shocked my doctor too. At this point, I had labored without medication for over 24 hours, and I was 100% done with it. I was frustrated, and since I knew I was just heading for another cesarean, I just wanted the contractions to go away.

My husband gave my doctor my gentle cesarean birth plan and he took it with him as he left the room. I was given medication to stop my contractions, and it was a relief. I was finally able to think more clearly. Everyone left the room. I sat on the edge of the bed, touching my belly where I knew my baby's head was settled, right under my heart, and cried. I didn't feel that I was strong enough. I thought we had at least one more week before our baby's birth day, but here I was about to have another C-section. We didn't even have a name.

My husband reassured me by saying he thought this was what was best for our son. He was right, but it didn't make the decision any easier. For nine months we couldn't agree on a name for our boy, and this was when my husband finally agreed on the name that I liked most. I'm not sure if it's because he wound up liking the name after all or if he felt sorry for me at that moment. He probably just didn't want us to have a nameless baby.

The anesthesiologist came into the room and explained the different types of medications she could use and gave me some options between a spinal or epidural as well as the pros and cons of each. I told her I didn't know what to do and she said it was okay, that I had time to think about it. I expressed my concerns over having low blood pressure every time I got the epidural and also wanting to avoid feeling drugged. She assured me that she would stay away from giving me narcotic medications if that's what I wanted. She also told me she read through my birth plan and said everything was doable and that she encouraged pictures being taken. I appreciated all the time she took to explain everything.

It wasn't long before the OR was set up and they were ready. Everything was calmer than I expected it would be. My feet hesitated to move as I stepped on to the operating table. As morbid as it sounds, it felt as if I was heading towards the gallows, that we were between life and death.

I really wanted to have my husband with me while they placed the spinal, but they told us he had to wait outside the OR. I had to go through this alone again. This was a source of major anxiety for my husband and I. It was especially so for him because he held onto the trauma of waiting outside the OR doors last time.

I was afraid, but I didn't want any drama. Even though he couldn't be right next to me, my husband sort of refused to leave the OR room and just stood in the doorway. It was kind of pointless because he refused to leave the room, but he couldn't be next to me. He watched with wide eyes as I screamed into the doctor's arms when they placed the spinal. I had so much back labor, I couldn't stand the feeling of the needle in my back. That was the worst part of the whole experience.

My husband came over and I felt his tears fall onto my face as he said he was sorry. I told him it was okay. I remember my breathing so vividly. Slowly I couldn't feel my belly, my legs, my feet, my toes. But I was still breathing. I watched my belly rise and fall with my breath until the curtain was up and I couldn't anymore. Then I tried to hang on to the feeling of it rising and falling as everything else went numb. I focused on the light above me. I moved my hands and my arms because they were the only things I could move. My baby was okay. I was okay. I had to be okay because there was no turning back.

It was such a strange feeling, like I could fall asleep, and also like I could have a full blown panic attack at any moment. They gave me an oxygen mask. With my first, I couldn't wait to yank it off my face. This time I felt like I needed it. I decided that I wanted to see our baby come out, what was I thinking?

Before we knew it, the anesthesiologist lowered the drapes for us so that we could watch him be born. It was so crazy to see his butt, then his long legs, as they emerged from behind the drape. The doctors were having a little difficulty getting his shoulders and head out because he was close to my ribcage. I felt so much intense pressure! All of this was very eye opening to watch because if they struggled getting him out of a four inch incision, then trying to get him out the other way could have been disastrous.

They finally got him out and they showed us our baby while doing some delayed cord clamping. My doctor almost handed my bloody, vernix covered baby to me over the curtain right away, and I was too shocked to say or do anything. The other doctor mentioned it would be a good idea to clean him off first. That didn't take long, and I was able to hold my baby skin to skin while I was being stitched up. At that moment, I was extremely happy and felt that I actually gave birth this time around.

The doctors and anesthesiologist checked in with me every step of the way. I was so glad that I wasn't given any unnecessary medications that made me drowsy and feel drugged like last time. I was alert and felt pretty good overall. All of this helped me feel like an active participant during the birth. I really felt like we were cared for and that there was so much love in the OR.

While I was being stitched up, my doctor told me my uterine muscles were strong and that I would have been a good candidate for a VBAC this time if my baby was in a better position. The other doctor chimed in that they were able to find my original scar and used it this time, too. In a weird way, it was a relief to me that I only have one scar on my uterus instead of two.

Originally, a repeat cesarean was the last thing I wanted, but at the end of the day, I was thankful my baby was here. He got to pick his own birthday, which was so important to me. I also got to experience labor that I felt robbed of last time.

The funny thing is, my appointment with the doctor who had been willing to discuss breech VBAC was scheduled for the day after my baby decided to be born. All the events leading up to his birth were God's way of saying, "Nope, the VBAC you wanted so badly isn't meant to be." I needed to believe that I trusted my instincts and that God was protecting us that day.

I believe we needed to be in the hospital for this birth. Everyone showed love and support for us that day. We were so happy that the hospital staff helped meet everything on my birth plan and didn't rush us during the process. I was thankful to them for caring for us and supporting me by not pressuring me into a certain decision. I knew this was the right birth for him.

Making Meaning

Needless to say, I was very baffled and frustrated about the fact that I have now had two breech babies and two cesareans. With my first baby, I blamed her breech position on her spunky personality. This time around, I knew I did literally everything right to avoid it and he still wound up being breech. I blamed myself and my body more this time than my first. I really just wanted the choice to deliver my baby in the way I felt was best, which was why I advocated for a VBAC in the first place. Overall, I was happy about my experience but still upset about the automatic C-section that came along with having breech babies.

After having two breech babies in a row, I had to have answers. I needed to know why. My chiropractor said he was seeing more breech babies during the pandemic, which was interesting to me. I had my theories. Maybe it was stress or anxiety. It could have just been a fluke. Or maybe it was something structurally "wrong" with me. Being the emotional but logical person I am, I just wanted to understand the why behind it.

My doctor never saw anything abnormal with my uterus during either of my cesareans, but I was still curious. So I met with a specialist and scheduled a hysteroscopy to see if I had an abnormal shape to my uterus. I wasn't sure what to expect, but I thought it was just a more advanced ultrasound. Shortly before the procedure, I realized this was more invasive than I originally thought. I was nervous but I wasn't going to turn back now. I wanted answers, and this was one of the ways I could get them.

The doctor had me sit on the exam table. Then she inserted the speculum and put a tube through my cervix to fill my uterus with fluid. She explained everything every step of the way. I grabbed on to the sides of the bed to brace myself, but it wasn't as painful as I had anticipated. It just felt intense.

The doctor looked at the ultrasound screen and said, "Hmm I don't think it's a septum but it does look kind of heart-shaped." She pointed to the screen. I asked her, "Is it more arcuate?" (Meaning bow shaped or curved). I had done my own research on the uterine shapes beforehand. She looked at me and said, "Yeah, I think so. It's somewhat heart shaped, but it's very slight. It looks like it's just another variation of normal."

After it was over, the cramping felt like I was having labor contractions. I took a deep breath as the doctor said, "I think you could have a head down baby. I would be surprised if you go three for three!" This should have had me relieved, but deep down I know that if I have a third, they will also be breech. It's just a strong feeling I have. And that feeling brought on more research. Will I always have to have C-sections? Is my body just not made to give birth? I had to know if there were other options out there.

Even though my boy was already here, my search for a VBAC breech supportive provider continued. It was going to be so much harder now that I have had not one but two cesareans. I stumbled across a name in a Facebook group of all places. This lady stated, "I know someone who would do it. I definitely suggest you contact him." She gave me the name and email address of a doctor two hours away. I sent him an email shortly after explaining my situation, and to my surprise, he replied back 20 minutes later. He gave me his phone number and told me to call him any time to discuss it further.

Was I really going to bother a doctor who was probably busy with other patients? Surely he would not have given me his phone number if he didn't want me to call. When I called, I wasn't even sure what I was going to say. He answered, and I awkwardly introduced myself. I was straight to the point and said, "I have had two breech babies and two cesareans. I know my third baby will probably be breech as well. Do you do vaginal breech deliveries for people like me? I have never had a vaginal birth. Would that disqualify me or something?" I was trying not to ramble. The doctor said, "I have attended several vaginal breech deliveries as well as VBACs after multiple cesareans. There are certain criteria that have to be met."

From there, I flooded him with questions. How long have you been doing this? Isn't it against your hospital's policy? What about malpractice insurance? What are the risks? How many bad outcomes have you seen? My head was spinning, and I was baffled that a breech VBA2C might be an option for me some day.

This doctor spent over half an hour on the phone with me talking about the Term Breech Trial (a controlled study on breech delivery) and how vaginal breech birth was a dying art. He had 40 years of experience. He ended the call by saying, "Next time you're pregnant, you can come here and I will help you."

I hung up the phone and was in disbelief. There were so many emotions. It gave me hope that there was another option other than scheduling another cesarean or attempting a home birth. It also annoyed me that I finally found a vaginal breech supportive provider three months after I already had my son.

It's a relief knowing that I have choices if we do have another baby. That being said, if we ever come to that point I might make a different decision. One thing I've learned is that it's great to make a plan and be aware of your options. It's also okay to deviate from that plan. Right at this moment, it's almost impossible to know what decision I would make for future births. The most important thing I do know is that the choice will be mine.

The Lessons Learned

When I think back on my son's birth, it is evident that God played a hand in how everything happened that day. I felt that I followed my intuition by choosing to give birth in the hospital instead of attempting a home birth. Even though I felt empowered through my cesarean this time around, I still felt so many negative feelings towards my body. I felt that I was damaged or broken. I kept telling myself that it all happened for a reason.

Through processing my experience, I realized that giving birth taught me so many lessons about motherhood. There was a lesson on following my own intuition when other people's opinions were everywhere. I learned about standing up for my children in the face of profound opposition. I even learned that I can't always convince my children to do what I want them to do.

During my pregnancies, I desperately tried to control my babies' positioning while they were in the womb. It was only after the midwife told me to practice acceptance that I remembered that my babies are individuals. They knew how they needed to be born, and I had to trust them. This has been one of the biggest lessons I carried into motherhood.

My children will make their own choices in life, some I may not agree with. No matter how much I teach them or try to guide them, I cannot control them. Our birth experiences can teach us so many things. This is why birth matters.

It's truly amazing what we can do for our children. When we become parents, we find a strength within us that we didn't know we had. For me personally, having another C-section was something I was very afraid of. I was afraid of the impact it would have on my baby, my health and future pregnancies. I was afraid of the needles, of the surgery, of all of it. I was even afraid I could die. I was afraid of these things, but I did it anyway.

I was determined and fought for a VBAC but still had a cesarean. I still had to overcome many things. I had to overcome doubt. I had to overcome my fear of conflict, especially when advocating for what was best for us. I had to overcome grief as I let the birth plan I wanted so badly go. One of the biggest things I had to overcome was my fear of another cesarean.

Even after all of that, the very thing I was so afraid of wound up being a beautiful and positive experience. This was the birth of my baby after all. When we previously think, "I could never do that," and we prove ourselves wrong, it's a powerful thing.

Birth of the Book

As part of processing my experience, I decided to tell my story to anybody who would listen. First I shared it on my doula page on Facebook among friends. Then someone reached out to me and asked if I would be willing to share on their blog. I was thrilled that somebody wanted to put my story out there.

The night my story was posted, the blogger called me and asked if I saw the first comment. I was a little taken aback. She warned me that it was negative and she had never had anyone react this way to any of the birth stories. Of course, I was nervous to read it.

It was a comment from a high risk labor nurse, and she was angry. She started off calling my story selfish and uninspiring. She said she could not get behind this "poor me" story because it seemed that I cared more about my birth experiences than my baby's well-being. She ended it by saying stories like these were the reason that women do dangerous things to achieve the birth they desire.

It was devastating for me to read. I felt that she missed the point of my story entirely, so I responded back. I told her she was right, that women are doing dangerous things to achieve the birth experiences they desired, which was the reason I shared my story. This is why I felt it was important for women to be presented options on how they wanted to deliver their babies. I told her, "Cesareans were not what I wanted. I have a right to be sad over that and still acknowledge that they were surgeries that brought my babies here safely."

The second time I shared my story was through ICAN for CBAC Awareness month. I was so excited to see that my story was selected to be shared on their Facebook page with over 60,000 people. Then I saw the very first comment, "This just makes me sad. She was lied to, her body was working. She should have just stayed home. Breech isn't a reason for a C-section."

Again, my heart dropped. Another negative comment but on the opposite end of the spectrum. Apparently I didn't try hard enough now. I responded back, "I educated myself on breech birth and I made the decision to have a repeat cesarean on my own. I felt this was the safest option. Things didn't line up the way I had hoped. However, I am not a victim here and should not be made to feel ashamed for my decisions."

I was so confused. On one hand, I had someone telling me I shouldn't be sad and I shouldn't have tried for a breech VBAC. On the other hand, I had someone else feeling sorry for me and telling me I didn't try hard enough. For whatever reason, my story and breech presentation stirred up a lot of strong emotions in people.

While it made me nervous to share my story, I knew I needed to do it and speak my truth. In doing so, I found that I wasn't the only one who was affected by the lack of options when it came to delivering a breech baby. Maybe I wasn't entirely crazy for feeling both happy and sad over my experience. It is real grief that can coexist with the joy I feel for my children.

One day, I was talking with some friends over a group chat on social media. One of my friends had recently found out she was pregnant. So naturally, the topic turned to pregnancy and birth. We talked about all our feelings, good and bad.

Some of them were ecstatic to find out they were pregnant, while others felt scared, sad or even angry when they saw that positive pregnancy test. That's when I realized how much shame we feel over our emotions. We can find validation and acceptance in each other's stories. There is so much that can be normal, and knowing we aren't alone can be healing. That is when I began thinking about writing this book.

Even when this book was already in the making, part of me thought, "Maybe I should wait a couple of years and see if I can have a natural birth. Then my story will really be inspiring." But then I realized that was part of the problem; there is still a stigma on cesarean birth, and there shouldn't be. As a doula, I felt like I had to prove myself. I felt embarrassed that I couldn't have a VBAC. It took some time to realize that I didn't have to prove anything.

If I felt so "unworthy" to share my story, did other moms feel the same way? What about other moms who had traumatic birth experiences? Are they also afraid to be open and honest about their birth stories?

I knew I had to make meaning from my experience. I may never have another baby, but starting this book made it feel like I was preparing for another birth. There was a lot of thought and planning put into this book. It was going to take time. It was painful to re-visit and write about some parts of my past. I felt like the guardian of all the stories so many others had entrusted me with. The thought of bringing it into the world was scary.

This is just a little bit of my story and the inspiration behind this book. In the process of gathering these stories, I realized there was a common theme: We are often afraid to share how we really feel. When we are told, "At least you have a healthy baby," and, "It doesn't matter how your baby is born," we tend to want to keep our feelings to ourselves. I encourage you to be open and honest. We do each other a great disservice by keeping silent. There are many others out there who are feeling just as you are. You are not alone.

Conclusion

So many of these stories could fit into more than one chapter or category. Every person and their story is beautifully unique. Every birth is beautiful, complicated, traumatic and powerful in its own way. I'm no one special, I just felt called to tell my story. This calling was strengthened as more mothers started sharing their stories with me. This just goes to show that birth is not just a one time event. We will always remember our children's birth days and how we were made to feel. These experiences affect our overall wellbeing. As parents we deserve to feel healthy, both physically and emotionally, so that we can take care of our little ones. We deserve more than just mere survival. In this day and age especially, we deserve to feel heard and supported.

Common Abbreviations
A Quick Reference Guide

AFE - Amniotic Fluid Embolism
AROM - Artificial Rupture of Membranes
CBAC - Cesarean Birth After Cesarean
CNM - Certified Nurse Midwife
CPM - Certified Professional Midwife
CPR - Cardiopulmonary Resuscitation
D&C -Dilation and Curettage
DO - Doctor of Osteopathic Medicine
ECV- External Cephalic Version
EDD - Estimated Due Date
ER - Emergency Room
GD -Gestational Diabetes
HBAC- Home Birth After Cesarean
HELLP - Hemolysis, Elevated Liver enzymes, Low Platelet count
HG - Hyperemesis Gravidarum
ICAN - International Cesarean Awareness Network
IUGR - Intrauterine Growth Restriction
MD - Doctor of Medicine
MFM - Maternal-Fetal Medicine
OR - Operating Room
OT -Occupational Therapy
PP - Postpartum
PPA - Postpartum Anxiety
PPD- Postpartum Depression
PPH - Postpartum Hemorrhage
PROM- Premature Rupture of Membranes
PT -Physical Therapy
RCS - Repeat Cesarean Section
ROM- Rupture of Membranes
TOLAC - Trial Of Labor After Cesarean
TTC - Trying To Conceive
VBB - Vaginal Breech Birth
VBAC -Vaginal Birth After Cesarean
VBAMC - Vaginal Birth After Multiple Cesareans (Other examples: VBA2C - Vaginal birth after two cesareans, VBA3C - vaginal birth after three cesareans, etc.)

Organizations and Additional Resources

American College of Obstetricians and Gynecologists (ACOG): acog.org
Amniotic Fluid Embolism Foundation: afesupport.org
Association for Prenatal and Perinatal Psychology and Health (APPPAH): birthpsychology.com
Birth Monopoly: birthmonopoly.com
Birth & Trauma Support Center: birthandtraumasupportcenter.org
Breech Without Borders: breechwithoutborders.org
Conquering CHD: conqueringchd.org
Hyperemesis Education & Research - HER Foundation: hyperemesis.org
ImprovingBirth: improvingbirth.org
International Cesarean Awareness Network (ICAN): ican-online.org
La Leche League: llli.org
Moms With Femoral/ Peroneal/ Sciatic Nerve Damage from Labor/ Delivery: nervedamagefromchildbirth.com
National Accreta Foundation: preventaccreta.org
NICU Helping Hands: nicuhelpinghands.org/resources
National Organization for Rare Disorders (NORD): rarediseases.org
Postpartum Support International: postpartum.net
Help Line: 1-800-944-4773
Preeclampsia Foundation: preeclampsia.org
Pregnancy After Loss Support: pregnancyafterlosssupport.org
RESOLVE: The National Infertility Association: resolve.org
Sexual Abuse Hotline: rainn.org
Help Line: 1-800-656-HOPE
Spinning Babies: spinningbabies.com
Stillbirthday: stillbirthday.com
Suicide Prevention Lifeline: suicidepreventionlifeline.org
Help Line: 1-800-273-TALK

Acknowledgements

I would like to thank "my village." To my husband, thank you for being a constant support and listening ear when I needed it. You were always there for me when I doubted myself, and your encouraging words helped keep me going.

To my mom, thank you for your never ending guidance. You were always there for me to offer advice and suggestions (even at strange hours of the night). I could not have done this without your support.

Thank you Christina, for spending countless hours editing, reading, and rereading the stories to correct grammatical errors, and for helping with the layout. I would be completely lost without your expertise.

Thank you Deborah, for making this beautiful painting for my book cover, formatting and praying over this book. Your support means the world to me.

To my friends, thank you for your constant support, and for giving me the idea for this book in the first place. Your advice and encouragement on this journey were so valuable.

Finally, thank you to all of the brave parents who contributed a story. I hope you feel heard, validated, and know that you are all worthy. None of this would be possible without you!

About The Author

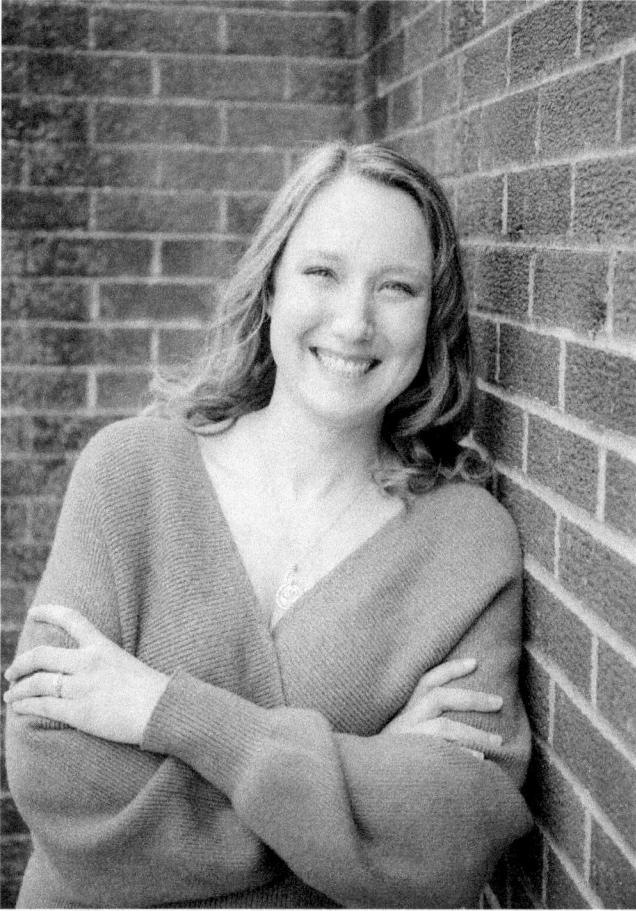

Kinsey lives in a small town in Iowa with her husband and two children. She became a certified birth and bereavement doula in 2016. She has a passion for VBAC, breech babies, and parents' rights during childbirth.

Variations of Normal is her first book.

www.ingramcontent.com/pod-product-compliance
Lightning Source LLC
LaVergne TN
LVHW051410080426
835508LV00022B/3014